F.I. ONE

F.I. ONE

MEMOIRS OF A FORENSIC INVESTIGATOR

JACK V. STURIANO

UNIFORM

This edition first published by Uniform in 2019
an imprint of Unicorn Publishing Group

Unicorn Publishing Group
5 Newburgh Street
London W1F 7RG

www.unicornpublishing.org

ISBN 978-1-912690-30-5

Printed and bound in Great Britain

Cover design by Unicorn
Book design by Vivian@Bookscribe

CONTENTS

*'To the button and the banana
and my cosmic gift'*

JOB DESCRIPTION

An employee in this class conducts independent and confidential investigations of deaths resulting from natural, accidental, criminal, suspicious and undetermined causes.

The investigator interviews witnesses, records detailed observations of the scene, takes photographs, collects evidence and reviews physician and hospital records.

Investigations are performed to obtain factual history and record of events with emphasis on manner and circumstance of death.

PERSONAL QUALITIES

Ability to deal sympathetically and objectively with people under stress, good judgement and persistence are deemed essential for the demands of this position.

PREFACE

Wilfred Owen wrote the preface for a poetry book before he had enough poems for that book; something he never published because of his death seven days before World War I ended. What's remembered about that preface is that he said, 'The poetry is in the pity'.

This is not a book of poetry, although there are some poems at the end. I have borrowed Owen's idea because the power of these stories is in the 'pity'. Each of these stories has a completely separate version sitting in a file cabinet in the medical examiner's office where I worked. They have narrative, minus adverbs, adjectives or emotion. They are written in medical-ese, like the average medical history with the physical exam on the back. The last thing that is wanted, or even spoken of, in medicine – is 'EMOTION'. It's not that there isn't plenty of emotion; it's just not good form to refer to it or, God forbid, to express it yourself. You dryly report your findings on paper or in person to doctors, and you're done. Medicine in America has now bred two or three generations of heartless practitioners by weeding out all 'emotion' by the simple expedient of only allowing people with high grade point averages to be admitted to medical schools. You want a doctor with a heart. The doctor with a heart will come out at two in the morning; the doctor with the high grade point average won't.

So what I have done is gone back in my memory and written

in the 'emotion' I could never, or was never allowed to, express. I am surprised at how much of it is still floating around in my psyche; but you will be the judge of this. I have added things that I wished had been said about the work we did, not only to each other but to the powers that be. It's not that we didn't say these things privately to each other, to doctors or to cops who were friends, but, being civil servants, knew what lines could not be crossed.

This work is a memoir but, like all memoirs, especially after a long life, things get distorted as to facts, events, persons, attitudes, and just plain forgetfulness. Most events in this memoir are close to forty years in the past and are not to be thought of in modern day terms. Things were radically different. It's almost ancient history and forensic medicine wasn't an exact science as it had only emerged about a decade before I arrived on the scene. When we told the boss that we knew nothing about forensic medicine, he tossed us a book on the subject and said if we had any problems at all to call him. That was it. It seems laughable now but terrifying at the time. It was a pre-computer, internet, cell phone, DNA age; not exactly halcyon days but fondly remembered. This memoir is under no obligation to be history. The best I shot for was honesty and feeling those emotions that at the time I couldn't dare give into but swore to myself I'd write about some day and that day has come. ENJOY.

THE HAIRCUT

I was dozing in the straight-backed wooden chair in old Mr Pelosi's barber shop. He was just finishing cutting the hair of a guy who was coughing up gobs of sputum into tissues that he pulled from a big box on his lap. The guy would almost strangle trying to cough this stuff up, but finally, with his face turning blue, the sputum would release its near-fatal grip on the lower reaches of his bronchial tree and be propelled onto the tissue, while Mr Pelosi waited; just this 'lunger', then the kid, then me, I thought.

The tattered copy of *Esquire* on my lap was a year old and missing the last page of the article I had started to read. I glanced towards the magazine rack but others were of similar age and condition. My eyes closed again. Mr Pelosi had gotten noticeably older in the past year. He had lost much of the flesh from his face. His once ruddy cheeks had been replaced with the gray, lifeless jowls seen in advanced cases of atherosclerosis. He hadn't shaved today; an ominous sign, I thought, when a barber doesn't shave. He still carried too much weight from the neck down, and his white smock was stained at just the point where food would hit his protuberant abdomen if it missed his mouth.

I took a look at his surgical jar with the blue disinfectant solution. It seemed the number of combs in the jar had been decreasing in direct proportion to the years I'd been coming to his shop. The jar was empty. He was on his last comb. It occurred to me that there was a good chance that he probably wouldn't be here the next time I came for my semi-annual beard trim and two-minute run of the scissors through what was left of my hair.

I silently cursed again the medical education that gave me these insights. I began to mourn for the old man whom I had grown to like as much for his warmth and humor as for the refuge his shop offered from the unisex, blow-dry, hairspray places that had taken over in our town in recent years.

I think the thing that originally attracted me to his shop was that it seemed as if it hadn't changed since it opened in 1949. When I passed the big barber pole swirling inside his shop, I would be entering a time warp, and suddenly it was 1955 and not 1987. I would be eight years old again, sent for my monthly 35 cent 'regular' haircut and the liberal application of the 'green stuff' that kept my hair in a perfect hardened cast for at least four days. The shelves were filled with bottles of various hair lotions and creams. There would be the poster of 'Fearless Fosdick' with bullet holes for Wild Root Cream Oil. Florida water, witch hazel, Bay Rum, hot towels, straight razor shaves, talcum powder in a cloud about your head. In the summer, my father would have us get crew cuts, but they were more like boot-camp cuts. Now all of these familiar male grooming rituals are all gone, and Mr Pelosi's shop just had some of this and it felt right. I still use Bay Rum.

I'm mourning not only Mr Pelosi's getting older and nearer to death but also my own lost youth. I see these signs all the time as a death investigator, and I just wish I could turn it off from time to time.

The 'Lunger's' haircut was finally finished. He gathered up his tissues and lit up a 'Lucky Strike', which brought on a paroxysm of coughing. Unable to speak, but waving goodbye, he left. It was the kid's turn and she was prompted toward the chair by one of a pair of elderly ladies who had been conversing just before with Irish accents. She was a small child with long, straight, black hair. She couldn't have been more than four years old and this was probably her first professional haircut. The girl was looking at Mr Pelosi with sad, fearful eyes, but his smiling face seemed to win her over. He very formally shook her hand and then shakily lifted her onto the child's seat and snapped the cloth around her neck. She looked warily at Mr Pelosi as he began to cut her hair.

My eyes began to close again and I wondered what it would be like to sleep for eight uninterrupted hours a night. The past forty-eight hours had been particularly brutal, if that term had any meaning left after the thousands of deaths I've seen in nine years. This last wave of death descended with tornado-like swiftness after a week that had been remarkable only for the vicious homicide of a young woman three nights before. Car and train accidents, drownings, hangings, cancer patients, had all arrived in a deluge of death. All this and the moon hadn't been full nor had there been any change in the weather or an approaching holiday – the usual harbingers of this much death. How much can a man take and still be part of the human race, I thought again.

I barely heard the little girl when she spoke. 'My Mommy died,' she said. Mr Pelosi turned to the two Irish ladies for help, and the little girl swiveled her head around to look at them. They remained mute with the same pained expression that Mr Pelosi wore. The little girl looked to the old ladies for some answer as to why her mother was dead, but seeing none, she turned back. Then one of the old ladies opened a newspaper behind the girl's back and pointed to the headline: 'SEARCH STILL ON FOR KILLER'. She rapidly waved her hand to signify that Mr Pelosi should drop the subject. Mr Pelosi said to the girl, 'I'm sorry to hear that'. Grim-faced, he continued to cut her hair. He didn't say anything when I walked out the door. When I returned the next day he didn't mention my abrupt exit and he did not mention the girl. It seemed we both looked grayer in the mirror and I had a hell of a hangover.

I never told him that I had pronounced that little girl's mother dead four nights before, because I couldn't believe it, didn't want to believe what I saw in that little girl's face. She had the same black hair, being cut as short as her dead mother's, and the same questioning look on her face as her mother's corpse.

PROPHECY ON HOTEL WALL

I got to the scene late. When you are the only F.I. on duty in a county of 1.5 million, it's going to happen, but not as often as you would think. Most everything was done.

This particular scene was in a chain hotel of repute, the only one in the county, and it went out of its way to make sure you knew it was an old-fashioned hotel and not a motel; but it was just an expensive version of our local 'hot sheet' motels. I have been in most of them at one time or another; most, I could find in my sleep. My favorite was the Sayonara Motel.

The man had checked in the day before and was currently residing in the bathtub filled with water, and half a dozen pill bottles nearby on the counter. Empty. I just had to examine the body and in a full tub it was easy, thanks to Archimedes. It seemed that I would probably get out quickly and on to my next case, but as I left the bathroom there was written on the bedroom wall in large letters 'Appointment in Samarra ...'

We always look for suicide notes and as it turns out this was a suicide note because *Appointment in Samarra* is the title of the first novel by a once famous doctor's son named John O'Hara, now completely forgotten. The protagonist in the novel commits suicide by driving his car into a garage with the engine running and shuts the door.

The book has a curious front piece of an apocryphal tale set in mists of antiquity which starts: Death Speaks. It seems a servant of a rich merchant was out in the market place of old Baghdad and meets Death in the guise of an old woman who makes a threatening gesture to him. Fearful, he rushes home to his master and begs to be given a horse to ride to Samarra to avoid his fate in Baghdad. After the servant gallops away the merchant returns to the marketplace and confronts Death who denies threatening the servant but admits being surprised by seeing the servant because she has an appointment with him in Samarra tonight.

The more I thought about this story, the more I was reminded of how, when I was in Vietnam serving as a Navy Hospital Corpsman with the 1st Marine Division in 1968, we used to have a saying: 'You sweat it, you get it'. This was the wisdom of the 'Grunts' who knew that whenever you felt (and we all did) that the next patrol, or ambush or road sweep, would be your last, some would be so spooked they would try to get out of doing it by feigning illness or trying to change places with others, or in extreme cases shooting hands, feet or head. I can't say these avoiders or worriers had a greater death rate but I did hear of a marine lance corporal who shot off his trigger fingertip, thinking they would send him home – but the Marine Corps decided he could pull the trigger with what was left and sent him back and he was killed shortly after. It was common knowledge that anyone who went back to the States on R&R would never make it home after, as happened to a marine who did this in another company. It's also true, in my opinion, that we had more casualties among married men with kids, and that marines and corpsmen with no one at all came through better. I think all these avoiding actions testify to something in men or life, that you pretty much seal your fate by certain courses of action and thought. I felt I would never come home alive from Vietnam, yet I did. That idea gave me comfort, it let me sleep by believing it. I came very close three times, yet I escaped, but there was always that fear and always the temptation to resist by going to Samarra (running away). That's what I learned in Vietnam: to control fear. It's not easy: it starts by being able to control the panic of facing death long before the shooting starts.

Now, if our servant had been able to see death and not panic (we are all going to die some day) and went home and stayed in Baghdad, he would have missed his fate in Samarra. I think the part I liked best about this story, and the part that few get, is that Death didn't know the servant was in Baghdad.

GETTING A-HEAD

The case is tossed on my desk by our petulant office secretary, with her usual bored flip of the wrist and her annoyed facial expression. My malevolent glare has no effect on her institutional nonchalance. I read the two lines which are characteristic of the usual wealth of information – Four heads, local dump, human or not.

I should call and get better information but it's not worth the aggravation, so I just close my eyes and sigh at what I have gotten already. I've had to visit scenes of various horrors, from dismembered bodies under trains to fly-covered corpses in the woods, in order to earn my daily bread in this Forensic Investigation business. It's getting to be one of those days when I curse my wish to even be in medicine. I should have stayed in the Navy. I'd probably be a Chief Petty Officer by now, on some nice little ship, air conditioned sick-bay, on a Mediterranean cruise. Forensic textbook in hand (I slept through the class on Forensic Anthropology) and my usual post-lunch indigestion starting to rise, I depart.

Three smokes and two wrong turns later, I arrive in the vicinity of the dump, unfortunately downwind. The road resembles one I saw in Quang Nam Province, Vietnam.

The crater to road ratio was definitely on the crater side. Undaunted, since I'm driving a county car, I proceed. I reach a shack where three gate guards sit with their feet up (at time and a half). They point me in the general direction of my goal, which is at the top of a small Mount Everest of garbage. The truck path to the top is a muddy track that I'm sure will swallow, whole, county cars. I decide to risk a fatal cardiac event and set off on foot. After all, my life is well insured and, more importantly, I am assured a ride back to the office if I leave the county car at the bottom of the mountain.

Shoes mired in unspeakable gunk, out of breath, and with a tachycardia of 180, I arrive at the top. There I find two foremen and one cop who had called it in and one million seagulls diving about à la Hitchcock. Sure enough, there are four nicely preserved human heads. I didn't need the textbook to figure it out. Nicely preserved doesn't mean intact though, as two of the heads have been cut in half – one vertically and the other horizontally – by a saw. They're fully fleshed, but brown from being what they are: anatomical specimens from an earlier age. They had been in a small garbage can of formalin which had been dumped sometime before by a man hired to clean out the office of an elderly physician who had died recently. This dump we are in is not too far from one of our county's huge mental hospitals, now almost all shut down. This doctor's office was in the same town.

In addition to the heads there are two dozen human

ears embedded in plaster, many with unusual shapes and deformities. The shapes of patients' ears used to be seen as part and parcel of congenital syndromes and mental illness. They also used to examine bumps on the head, something called phrenology, which was big at one time in medicine but, much like blood letting and leeches, has had its day. There were also some great volumes on medicine in leather covers. *Osler's Modern Medicine* – all twelve volumes – and a book I kept: *Electricity in Ear, Nose and Throat Disease*, and medical journals which, along with the rest, should have gone to some medical library. There were some instruments in an old-fashioned table boiler, now sadly rusted and corroded, but just looking at them made me glad I lived in an age with modern anesthesia and pain techniques.

So, added altogether, it seems our doctor had some training aides from an earlier age. This was later confirmed by a phone call to his widow and one old doc in our office who knew him in his youth.

I gather up these heads and ears and head back downhill as the seagulls seem to be heading in for the kill, secure in the knowledge that downhill is easier than uphill. 'You have to climb a mountain sometimes if you want to get a-head in this business – hahahahahaha...'

THE RUSSIANS

The thing I love about this job is the sheer fucking randomness of my crazy days. It's like the enjoyment of a nice air strike on a tree line. There is something horrific but satisfying when I'm in this mood.

Just when I think it can't get any stranger, gruesome, sick, disgusting, sad, and a couple of other adjectives and adverbs and a few exclamation points, then, as Travis Bickle says in *Taxi Driver*, 'Days go on and on and then there is change'. It's a routine day on call (overtime) as usual.

It's late Sunday afternoon and I've made some overtime money and not worked hard for it, when I get the call. It's in a quiet neighborhood where I haven't been for some time, but it's next to another neighborhood where I have cases all the time for some reason, and I'm wondering about all this as I drive down. It's a small wooden house, a converted bungalow. I walk in. I'm confronted by a weird sight and smell. In the living room and adjacent smaller room are empty cages, big cages, stacked about six feet high, about two dozen, each about three feet wide by three feet tall. The smell is of something feral but subdued by Lysol. I look at the cop. He says the precinct got a call from a friend of the deceased. It's a lady who hasn't shown up for church on Sunday. It turns out she is Russian, from a tight-knit group of recent immigrants. 'So where is the body?' I ask. 'In the bathroom,' he says. I shouldn't have asked as they are almost always in the bathroom and it's hard to move them around and examine them, but that's what I get paid for.

Now, as I said, every time you think you've seen it all... well, anyway, this woman is in the bathtub and she is boiled like a chicken in a pot. I got this later from a relative but it seems she would take a bath once a week on Saturday nights (we used to do the same in the '50s when I was a kid). She liked a hot tub and would get in and soak to be ready for church on Sunday. She would just crack the hot water faucet with her toes when the water cooled off to keep it hot. What she died of is unknown. She was seventy-nine and had a bad heart. It wasn't drowning, as her head was out of the water. Let's just say that her autopsy was inconclusive, as are most with heart disease. The Japanese bathe in water very hot, but never let water above heart level. Good idea. The problem here is that this toe business has led to a situation where the water in the tub was still hot when I got there. How hot? Well, I didn't have my thermometer but I yanked a small one off a calendar from the Russian Orthodox church (crude but effective) and it said 118 degrees. Seems that her water heater was set at 180 degrees for her dishwasher rinse cycle, so by just letting a trickle of water into the tub, the water heater was able to keep up with the loss.

Now you may not know this, but once you're dead you become the temperature of the environment you're in, so she was being slowly par-boiled like a chicken in a crockpot on a low setting, and it's not pretty and the aroma of boiled human is not pleasant. A cursory exam showed that, like most boiled things in a pot, moving them around or pulling an arm or leg leads to... well, let's just say, to 'problems'. Getting her out of the tub would lead to visions imprinted on your synapses which, trust me, you will never be able to forget. I knew one thing for sure, I didn't want to be around when the morgue guys showed up to get this body. How did I know this? I learned it in college. The University of Danang, class of 1969. I majored in medical repairs, but I had a minor in the use of the POUCH/HUMAN REMAINS/ 1A/ COMBAT INDIVIDUAL/OD. We had a rifle team and they were pretty good. You may have heard of them: the United States Marine Corps. We were involved in those years in the Great Southeast Asia war games. The games lasted a long time – from 1965 to 1971. We came in second place. They had more targets than we had.

So I went and spoke to the cop but delayed calling for the wagon. I started looking around the rest of the house as I was now curious to find out what the Russian lady kept in the cages. The other rooms gave no clue. These converted bungalows have no second floor but deep basements. Finding the door, I open it but the light switch is not working.

It's pitch black below but I can see the landing from the light, let in from the door. Neither the cop nor I has a flashlight. I have lost dozens and won't buy another; so has the cop.

When I got to the bottom I turned around and almost had a heart attack. I was immediately confronted with the scariest thing I've ever seen on this planet. There was just enough door light to illuminate forty sets of eyeballs peering out of the dark at me. Big, bright, luminous eyes, staring like some thousand-eyed creature. I think I actually felt the hair rise on my head, though I'm bald! I yelled up to the cop to open the door wider and then I could see that there were cages filled with cats. Not just any old cats, but Persian blues. Big heads, wide-set eyes and, even weirder, they were mute. They never made a sound. Their mouths opened as if to make a sound but not a peep. They just stared from their cages. Why they were in the basement in the dark I'll never know. I told the cop to call the town animal shelter to come and get them and the wagon and I got out of there as fast as I could.

The morgue wagon drivers still talk about this woman, when they try to top each other on terrible cases they have had to pick up. Curiously, this is the second famous Russian our office has had. Back in the early '70s, before I started, some fisherman trawling with big bottom rigs had trawled up a Russian corpse which had been buried at sea. The body was wrapped in canvas, had Russian boots and a big 'Y' incision of autopsy across his front. The Russians had big fish factory ships off our coasts in those days. We advised the Russians of our find but they never responded. The body was kept in the old set of drawer-type refrigerators we had back then and was just left there when we switched to the big box refrigerators. He was mostly forgotten, but every now and then the cooling system for the old refrigerators would crap out and the Russian would make his presence known rather pungently and repairs would be made very quickly. At some point, maybe twenty years later, they paid some funeral home to take the body away and bury it in an unmarked grave. Where you're born and where you die; therein lies the tale.

SUICIDE YEAR

I t was one of those weeks early in the new year when I began to realize it was going to be a suicide year for me. When you investigate deaths for a living you get yearly cycles of more of one kind than another. Last year was a MVA (motor vehicle accident) year for me. It seemed as if every other day or so I was pulling a body out of a car with those cracked skulls crunching under my hands, prying shattered limbs from under crushed dashboards or giving lessons in street anatomy (organs in the street), because a good many of these cases were pedestrian hit-and-runs and it was wearing me down. This was not my first suicide year. My first year at the office was a suicide year. There are patterns within this pattern, with firearms deaths predominating over, say, CO (carbon monoxide) deaths, or hangings over overdoses or train fatalities, and suicidal drowning was very popular one year for some reason.

This week I'd already had two suicides – a pistol shot to the head and a hanging. The hanging was the previous night and I was still somewhat numb from having to see a nine-year-old boy hanging in his closet. In all the hangings I'd had over the years no one had ever fashioned a hangman's noose. This boy had managed to fashion a classic 13-turn hangman's noose.

On a wall outside his closet was a plaque consisting of rope in various knots I'd last seen in the *Blue Jackets Manual*, when I was in the Navy. Bowlines, hitches, double carrick bends, cat's paws and a small hangman's noose, all very difficult to tie. I could never learn to tie them in the Navy yet this boy had learned to do so for a cub-scout badge. The boy killed himself because his parents had divorced two years earlier and he had lived with his mother after the separation. His mother had just died of cancer and he had come to live with his father and his new mother and siblings.

I'm thinking of all this as I drive to my next case. How is it possible that, in a twenty-four-hour day and a seven-day-a-week cycle, and me working thirty-five hours plus overtime, I still manage to be on duty when these cases occur or the body is found? Was it possible that I was attracting these cases?

I used to work for six surgeons as their assistant and the most amazing thing about them was that after a while I noticed that their patients were somehow linked to aspects of their personalities, good or bad. One surgeon, who I had actually met ten years earlier as his patient when he removed my appendix, was still always in a hurry to remove himself from every patient contact as soon as possible. He would breeze in, rip off the dressing, make a mess, and flee, leaving the sheets stained and nurses flinging curses at his retreating form. Invariably, once I got to know him and his patients, you could see that indeed his patients were the slowest people in speech and movement, and this drove him to a frenzy as he tried to keep his office schedule on track.

One other was an excellent but fussy surgeon who had these rituals he created for his patients to follow in their wound care. His patients were just as fussy if you had to care for them when he wasn't around or was away. My favorite was a sweet fellow with a heart of gold. His patients were the same but their illnesses made them much harder to deal with because they were so sweet and their illnesses so terrible, and they had all the worst complications to make it worse.

(I know the real reason that I'm getting these cases – hell, I was a neuropsychiatric technician in the Navy, but that's another story.)

It took me a while to find this house, but on arrival I was met at the door by the sector cop who told me that an old woman, who was not a family member but a close family friend, had been renting the basement apartment and had been found dead by the family, who hadn't heard from her in a day or so. The cop was having a nice time talking to the pretty daughter of the owner, but I interrupted to get a history of the usual medical problems and medications and something unusual. It seems this woman had not slept in the bedroom of the apartment since the death of her husband four years before. She had been sleeping on the couch in the living area. Now this is not as strange a story to an FI as it may sound. Many elderly people sleep in chairs or recliners because they can't lie flat due to failing lungs and hearts. I wondered why she was in the bedroom now, and as soon as I entered I knew. It was a small memorial to their lives together. Childless as they were, they had each other's love in full measure. She was lying on top of the satin bedspread. She was completely dressed as if she were going out on a date in 1950. Her make-up was perfect, her seams straight, and her hair in a style my mother wore in those days. She was on her side of the bed. She had been dead about two days. I had to move her around a bit to examine her, but she was still in rigor mortis so I was able to put her back in almost the same way. I went and found her pills, and I made a count and it confirmed what I saw in the bedroom.

As I was driving back, I knew this was going to be a suicide year because this old woman had committed suicide. It was a classic scene as described in all the forensic textbooks. The made-up bed, the best clothes, the elaborate make-up and hair, confirmed by a couple of dozen missing heart pills, just enough to kill someone with heart disease painlessly. These signs all said suicide.

When I thought about it later, what really got me was how she hadn't slept in that bed for four years since the death of her husband and had chosen to return to their bed in the end to be where he last was. It still gets me now in the throat when I think about it.

USUAL NIGHT

I ts 2:45 am and I have come to the only house on the block with the lights on and a cop car outside. Since the house has steep steps, through the picture window I can see only the heads of the people in the living room. To me, still only half-awake, these heads seem to float in the air. Hallucinations are a sign of sleep deprivation, but medicine wants its practitioners sleep-deprived – it maximizes profits. I blink a few times at the sight to try and clear my head.

I approach a screen door with a piece of rope for a handle. As I pull the door open, a large dog lunges at me and I wake up real fast. The dog is restrained from its zeal (aimed at my throat). After apologies for the dog and introductions by the cop, I see a plaque on the wall. It's a bronzed hammer that was awarded to the dead woman's son-in-law for being a good high school metal crafts teacher. This accounts for the do-it-yourself look to the house.

It is a routine case and, after I examine the elderly dead woman, I go to a nearby bathroom to wash my hands, a ritual that is being replaced by the use of vinyl gloves for most medical-human interactions. As I wash my hands, I'm reminded that I should carry gloves: still after twenty-plus years in medicine and nursing without using them in ordinary care, the practice just doesn't seem right. The only reason I'm in the home of these people whose mother has died of emphysema is because the woman's doctor didn't want to come and pronounce her dead. I don't know why he refused to come. I had asked him to take care of his patient but his incredulity at my request indicated he felt no obligation to come and pronounce his patient dead.

I don't know where I got the 'idea' that a doctor caring for a patient would be interested enough to attend the patient when she is lying dead on the floor of her room surrounded by the medicines and inhalators that he had prescribed for her. I think the 'idea' is called common decency and concern, but medicine seems to be short on this commodity in its practitioners these days. This dead woman is also surrounded by grieving loved ones and a police officer who won't let anyone touch the body, in case something is suspicious. The police officer is just doing his job and he's only here as well because this woman's doctor wouldn't get out of his bed to come, but if this family is like mine, a police officer has never been near, let alone inside, their home.

If my memory serves me, the Hippocratic Oath says something about the medical practitioner attending the patient under all circumstances. Why would that responsibility end with the patient's death?

In the old days (sixty years ago) when doctors came to

your home, they could actually do very little compared to modern techniques, but they came and sat at the bedside and examined and talked with the family and this is remembered as the Golden Age of Medicine – by patients, anyway. Simple human touching, concern and sharing. They could come, and pronouncing people dead is very simple, not high-tech, and most of what is done in the office they could do at your home very easily, but that wouldn't maximize profits as the average physician sees one patient every fifteen minutes today, hardly time to get undressed. Coming to a patient's home is very instructive for the physician. I once called a big professor of Pulmonary Medicine to tell him his patient had died. He told me that it was a difficult case and the patient never seemed to respond to treatment for her asthma. I said maybe it was because her room was filled with cat hair and dust because she never cleaned it. The carpet was literally white with hair and the rest of the house as well was an asthma nightmare. Now that I think of it my call to this doctor may have led him to recognize the value of a house call in this modern day. Unfortunately, this doctor's only recorded house visit was to his own home to murder his wife. Unlike doctors who hate to leave their ivory towers, my friends the detectives love to make visits anywhere.

Surely caring for patients has to involve more than giving medicines? Isn't the physician's role to share the anxiety, pain, suffering and degradation of some small portion of the diseases that we know so well and the patients and families so little? Shouldn't the physician comfort not only the patient but also concerned family members who have to watch their loved ones gradually lose the battle to age and disease? I was lucky, maybe too lucky, because early in my career I was acquainted with such physicians, and that's why I chose to be in health care, but it's been a long time since I've seen anyone who shares these sentiments, and none in the last ten years or so.

I do all the things the physician could have done. I lift her from the floor and cover her. She was very frail and thin; emphysema does that. I turned off the oxygen. The family and the police officer are grateful because she had been on the floor for a couple of hours and no one likes to see their loved ones like that. I've performed this act hundreds of times for physicians who just don't see this act as part of the modern practice of medicine. I'm sure this woman's doctor must wear gloves for every patient — but that's what's missing in this business of dealing with human beings – TOUCH. They need the touch of human contact as well as respect and courtesy as much as drugs, diagnoses and treatments.

On the way out, I pass the bronze hammer and reach for the rope door-handle. I guess I live in an age where shop teachers don't fix door handles but teach others how to, and doctors don't see their dead patients but have efficient billing services. I wonder again, but only briefly, about the order of things in the world. Why am I always on the wrong side of these issues in this profession I have chosen to make and have made my life's work?

FATHER AND SON

It's HOT!!! It's August and it's the worst month of the year for forensic work. It's when you get those long stretches of upper 80's and lower 90's. It's the kind of weather we had in Vietnam, when you wake up in the morning and your eyelids are sweating already. You also know that they are out there (floaters: decomposed bodies) waiting for you to come on duty. You silently pray you might possibly get away with it this day, but your enemy the FLY is doing his biological duty to make a normally pretty nasty bit of employment a million times worse – and I do mean a million.

I'm shortly to enter a room where a drunk has been keeping terminal company with a couple of hundred flies for a week or so. You know the type of flies, big and ugly with iridescent backs and about a million of their offspring. It took a week for the other residents to decide that the new odor was worse than the normal background smell of the place and investigate to find this man. I suspect it was not the smell as much as the fact that it is twenty days since social security checks came on the first of the month and they are looking for a bottle to share.

When I arrived, there was a fire truck and half a dozen firemen and cops standing around outside. Since I saw no smoke I knew what kind of case it was. I have had them before and will again. I refuse breathing devices because they fog up my glasses. The assembled firemen and cops are incredulous that anyone would enter such a room without such a device. Wearing their devices, they follow me in. There is a lot of buzzing and you have to make sure you keep your mouth shut. If you listen close enough you can hear it; the sound of all those little bites being taken all at once and repeatedly, or maybe it's just the sound of the writhing bodies. I examine the body just like any other physical exam, except you have to move the maggots over a little bit to look for signs of trauma. The hardest part is to make sure that our man has only the holes he was born with. The maggots make holes as well in places like the neck and face that, unless you have seen it before, can look very suspicious. The only thing worse (much worse) than missing a homicide case in this setting is to think one of these extra holes is homicidal and drag the forensic pathologist, crime lab people, photographers and detectives into this room to view your mistake.

Fortunately our man is lying on his bed and sheets make an excellent slide into the bag and the morgue wagon guys carry him out. I get the usual refrain from departing cops and firemen: 'I don't know what they are paying you but it's not enough to do this.' I smile. I get into the county car and of course the air conditioning isn't working and a few of those flies have followed me to the car; undaunted, I head back to the office.

As I drive, I think again of my father's line of work for all his years and I have to laugh. You could say that my father and I have the same line of work: dealing in end products. He was a sanitation man and I am a Forensic Investigator for a Medical Examiner.

We both worked nights. We both drove government vehicles. We both had routes, wore uniforms of sorts, and we both provided a service, a necessary one for the public. We were both called out after the society, of which we are part, recognizing that nothing else could be done with what is left, whether it was cherished, enjoyed, loved or abused, broken or worn out.

As a kid I always used to say, like most kids, that when I grew up I wanted to be just like him. He would say maybe I should try something else. He knew that he just took the sanitation job because after the war employment was hard to find and city jobs were middle-class gold. Still are.

I was ill with the measles and had to spend a week in a darkened room (something to do with the eyes). He told me stories about his work and the amazing things they would find in the garbage. They found money, rings, personal objects, and once a set of surgical instruments with bamboo handles in a bamboo case. He told me how they used to make extra money taking family pets to the dump, usually fifty cents or a dollar, and how for five dollars they would put the pet on the tailgate of the truck, put on their sanitation caps and drive it around the block for the family in a kind of funeral procession. He would tell me about the old Italian men who could hardly speak English who made up the bulk of the employees – like the cops, who were all Irish. He would talk about his Navy days in the Seabees on New Caledonia, Guadalcanal, and Guam, working twelve-hour days for three years unloading ships, but never how tough, brutal or dirty it must have been on hot August days.

Interestingly, these sanitation men, like my father, who were so physically active lifelong, all lived to advanced ages. They collected pensions in retirement that paid them three times what they had ever made in any year they worked when young men, and for longer than they had ever worked for the city.

I learned from my father a joy and wonderment at it all, even having to do life's dirty little jobs. I'll tell you a secret that he knew, I know and you now know. There is on this end of life's scale a freedom that you will never find in any other work situation. You are pretty much left alone by your employers and work finished quickly allows… well, let's just say, employee prerogatives are found. Charlie Parker, the saxophone giant, used to lay whole symphonies of music between whole musical notes of known standards. In this business you get to play between the notes like him.

My father was never morose or sad, and the only time I ever heard him complain was when it snowed and he knew he'd be gone for days having to plow the roads. It never ceases to amaze me how I wound up in this parallel universe to his, despite my fancy education. You know what, Pop? I got my wish. I'm glad and proud to follow you and be a man like you - except on hot August days.

BRING 'EM BACK JACK

It wasn't long after I started at the Medical Examiner's office, maybe a year or so, that I acquired the nickname 'Bring 'em Back Jack', awarded me by the morgue wagon drivers. It was meant as a mocking term for the fact that since my arrival they had to work harder, longer, and more often, bringing in bodies that had never had to come into the morgue. Maybe it was alliterative as my partner who proceeded me by a half year also brought in more bodies, but his name was Tom. Well you get the idea how the drivers felt about us. Tom and I were hired to replace a dozen or so police surgeons who, as a group, were pretty desultory in their forensic duties. They had one ability we did not have though; they could sign death certificates. So almost every case where we could not get an attending doctor to sign off the body had to come to the office to be examined.

With no such ability, and the fact that we were new to our roles as Forensic Investigators, we tended to err on bringing them in rather than signing them out. All to the drivers' disgust.

The Bring 'em Back Jack was based on a book by the famous American animal collector, Frank L. Buck – *Bring 'em Back Alive*. He collected animals from all over the world to bring back for zoos and circuses. He died in 1950 but his movie shorts were a staple of Saturday movie houses which I saw and later on TV.

Two guys go deer hunting during the short season in January in a wooded area of our county in an attempt to reduce the huge deer population which is overrunning the county and bringing high levels of Lyme disease from the ticks they carry as well as destroying expensive vegetation and gardens to feed themselves. You can only use shotguns not rifles. The shotguns take a huge metal slug, as they are called, but are actually bullets of large caliber similar to Minié ball of the American Civil War which is a .58 caliber bullet. The advantage in using these slugs is that they are powerful enough to kill but only at short distances. One hundred yards or less and in the woods more than likely if missing a deer it will hit a tree, not a citizen from a mile away like a rifle.

Now these two guys are a kid in his mid twenties and an older man in his mid forties who has never been deer hunting before but is a yearly duck hunter whose season has just ended in December. Having been an active duck hunter myself since the age of sixteen, I know that to shoot ducks by law your shotgun can only hold three shells even though the magazine can hold five. Usually a small wooden plug is inserted in the magazine to prevent more than three shells from being loaded.

In deer hunting you can use five slugs and conveniently they are sold in packs of five.

Now our duck hunter in this story has removed the plug and loaded in five slugs to his ancient Winchester Model 12 pump action shotgun, originally made with a shortened barrel for use by troops in the trenches in World War I. It was called the 'Trench Cleaner' because when used with double 00 shot it was a very effective weapon. It's been used in all of America's wars. We had Marines using them in Vietnam when I was there, mostly in ambush situations. Civilian use was just as popular with different barrel lengths, with extra long for Geese.

The younger man has been hunting deer before and has set up two tree stands to spot the deer. These stands can be climbed up, not to any great height, but it gets you above ground for better observation and off your feet.

So on a frosty morning at 6 am before sunrise, with snow still lying on the ground from a storm two days before, they set off into the woods. The plan is that they will hunt till noon and meet again in the parking lot. They separate from each other's effective range about a mile into the woods.

The young man says that at about 10 am he heard four shots in rapid succession followed by silence. When he heard no other sound or call from the older man he presumes that the shots missed. So at noon he walks back to the parking lot to await his companion who has the car keys. He waits almost two hours and then walks back to town which is some distance away. As the sun is going down, and after calling the older man's wife only to find that he has not returned home, he goes to the Police Dept.

The police hear the man's story but it takes them a while to get a search party together and consequently the body is not found till 11 pm. They also found four empty shotgun slug shells under the tree stand he was in.

I'm sitting warm and comfortable in the office reading, thinking so far so good. Only one case earlier, but it's bitter cold and I'm done in two hours, when I get the call. Now it takes us almost two hours to get to this location as our office is at the other end of the county. So now it's 1 am, my quitting time. It's a beautiful night and a full moon reflecting off the snow and stars at this end of the county is a beautiful sight. So off we go with snow crunching under our feet. One detective, two patrolmen, myself and my driver with a body bag. We all have big flashlights but it's a hike of some distance before we come to the body.

Our duck hunter is face down with his shotgun underneath him with the wooden stock missing. He also has a hole in the back of his hunting jacket. He's wearing so many clothes that it's hard to see anything deeper. At this point I don't know what I'm dealing with here but I know the wise play is to cover him with a tarp, set a police guard and come back in daylight. I tell this to the detective with the additional caveat that even now we may have stomped on critical evidence just being where we are. I also point out when the detective does not want to follow my advice, that the FBI manual states the same, but he still refuses. I'm not picking on this detective; at the other end of the county no one sits on a body till daylight.

I roll him over and sure enough he has a hole in the center of his chest near the bottom of his breastbone, on the same plane as the exit wound and it's not a contact wound. I notice that there are some coarse animal hairs on the body of the weapon. There is one empty shell in the chamber.

I say we should fan out in a 360-degree radius to see if we can find the wooden stock of the weapon. I have taken about twenty steps when sitting on the ground motionless, but with it's head erect, is a young buck deer with a huge wound to its posterior just above it's right leg, which is now congealed with blood.

My yell brings the rest running and we are stupefied to see this scene. Well, I was anyway.

The bright light has transfixed the deer, something that happens when hunting them at night and which is curiously known as 'Jacking', but it's starting to quiver a lot and is making a very feeble attempt to move but cannot.

So we got a dead duck hunter with an empty shell in his weapon, deer hair on the body of the weapon, no wooden stock and a young buck deer about 20 feet away. This is clearly a three pipe problem, as Sherlock would say, or time to get the little grey cells working as Poirot would say.

Since I'm me, I again say we should cover the body and leave, but I am again refused this option. Now it's clear the deer needs to be put down as it's suffering, so it's duly dispatched; unfortunately it takes four bullets from a .38 caliber pistol to do so. We had to make two trips to get the body and the deer back to the morgue. We never found the stock even when looking in daylight the next day.

In this State, at least since the fifties, in order to get a hunting license to hunt anything you have to take a Hunter's Safety Course. Basically, it does this by telling you the DO's and DON'Ts of hunting and handling weapons. Like, unload your weapon before climbing over fences. Wear red clothing and don't use white handkerchiefs as it may look like a white-tailed deer from a distance. Mostly it's a series of ghastly photos of people who didn't follow the rules. Not one of these photos was of a duck hunter, that's what I learned.

In this State in winter in deer season is filled with guys blasting away with 'Buck Fever' – the mania for the kill.

At the morgue, as you might imagine, Bring 'em Back Jack had finally earned his nickname causing much mirth in repeating it to me.

Theories abounded. Did the wounded deer attack the deer hunter? If so, why was it so far from the body? Yet the weapon had deer hair on it. The deer had a fair sized rack of antlers on its head. If he wounded the deer and obviously chased it, why didn't he shoot it with his remaining shell?

Autopsy sure enough reveals he was shot through the heart

with exit out the back. The deer has a slug in its hindquarters and four in its head. There is some gunshot residue on the front of his jack but it's not close.

I knew the answer and by getting my own shotgun, which was the same length as his weapon and both of us being approximate in height, I figured it out.

My hunting partner of many years, another Tom, was left handed and I'm right handed. So it was great in the duck blind and a lot safer. He too had an old Model 12 Winchester but after many years of use it was falling apart and he could fire it three times while holding down the trigger just by pumping it. You shouldn't be able to do that, but that's what happens. Some guys file down the sear to do just that. These guns are dangerous. Another friend failed to unload his Model 12 (State Hunter Safety Rule number 4) and laid it down in the bottom of his duck boat. As the boat hit the waves coming back the gun went off and blew a hole in the bottom of his boat. Fortunately he made it back home.

So the case it is 'SOLVED', as another famous detective once said. Our duck hunter confronts the deer which I feel was standing. He could of shot it but you see he's a duck hunter used to three-shot salvos. In his excitement (Buck Fever), he doesn't realize he still has a shell in the chamber, or maybe the deer charged him. Anyway, he grabs the shotgun by the muzzle and raises it over his head and brings it down in an arc and on impact it goes off. The arc it has to take is pure horizontal to get him through the heart. That's how the deer hairs got on the body. The stock went flying, never to be found, and those stocks can take a beating but indicates how powerful a blow it must have been. The deer had no other visible injury other than the shotgun wound.

There is always one unanswered question. Why didn't the young man hear the last shot? I believe the weapon went off so close to the man's body to muffle the sound enough.

I gave up hunting a few years back. I think about that man sometimes. He should have stuck with ducks.

MAN-O-MANISCHEWITZ

You really have no idea when you make a living as an investigator just how humdrum and routine lots of your work is until you get a case like this one.

We had had a particularly shitty winter. It seemed like every ten days or so we would get snow storms with sleet and freezing rain. Finally, after a rather late spring at the end of April, one night I get this case. I remember it was a Sunday and cold and dark. EMS had big arc lights up in this industrial park with lots of empty 'LOTS', waste ground, illegal dumps and abandoned cars. Seems some young boys had been playing in this location earlier before sunset. They were walking along a small berm of sand when they spotted a snake – a BIG snake. They went looking for a stick to poke it with and on the other side of the berm found a dead man lightly dressed with his shirt pulled up. The snow in this area had only disappeared a few days before. Sure enough the man was still frozen solid and had two very obvious fang marks on his lower abdomen.

The snake is huge, at least 6 feet, and very muscular. It is a nice orange-brown color with the classic diamond back pattern and a good size rattle which didn't as it was frozen as well. I got an evidence bag from the EMS guys, put the snake inside the bag and put it in the large pocket of my overcoat. The detectives didn't think this was a good idea as the snake could have been hibernating. I knew I was pretty safe as snakes can't tolerate weather like this and since it was in a plastic bag soon it would have no oxygen – because snakes breathe.

As it turns out the dead guy has ID in his pants and soon a police report with his name on it is found with the following series of events that led him to his place of death. It seems that in late February, during one of those howling weekly snow storms, our dead man has been living in the attic of a former girlfriend who has taken him in after his exotic pet business has folded and he has no place to live. Her new boyfriend makes enough for them to rent an older house with lots of rooms. I know this place he used to own as it was on a major highway close to a train bridge which I used to pass regularly. Exotic pets is a code word for poisonous and it means snakes, spiders, ferrets, etc.

Things are going fine until one day he gets amorous with his ex. She manages to fight him off and get to a phone; he immediately ceases any further attempts and heads upstairs.

No sooner does she put the phone down than our would be former exotic pet shop owner comes raging down the stairs with a huge rattlesnake in both hands, held over his head, doing what it does when it is pissed off – RATTLE.

Off he goes into the night in a howling blizzard. The policeman who took the report, I am certain was not convinced of its veracity, which is a mild way of saying what they really thought. It was a busy night in snow storms with lots of fender benders.

As it turns out this industrial park is not far from the place where he was staying with his old girlfriend. About a mile away. The snake turns out to be probably the most poisonous snake in the USA; it's a Mojave desert rattler. It bites about 600 people a year and kills about eighty, or so the authorities in Arizona inform us.

Since the body was frozen it needed to be warmed up to do an autopsy. That's done by leaving it in a heated hallway for a day. Unfortunately snake venom is organic and disappears on defrosting. My question is, when did the snake bite him? He was able to travel a mile or so and the snake is about 20 feet away from his body before cold stopped it, so it must have been alive.

So there it is, the story of how 'Bring 'em Back Jack earned his nickname years after he got it. God I love this job.

INGENUITY

'Among the common run of men there are many of little personality and stamped with no deep impress of fate, who find their end in suicide', *Treatise on the Steppenwolf* by Herman Hesse.

Old H.H. and I know a thing or two about suicide. I read Steppenwolf at least once every year or so, especially when it was a slow night at the morgue. He has a lot more to say about suicide but it's about sensitive types: like Herman and me. I don't see many of those in my line of work. Mostly those of 'no deep impress and little personality', who in their suicides have certainly impressed me as few other cases I have had. This story is almost as strange as the corpse.

It's late afternoon, a weekday, about 4 pm. The fire department gets a call to a fire. They arrive, but find no fire, just a strong smell of something burnt, a slight haze to the air, and a dead guy near the boiler in his basement. Even weirder, the family tells the cops that at about 2 pm a man had knocked at their front door, introduced himself and said he was the new owner of the house. He had bought the house from the bank, which had sold it because the mortgage had not been paid in a year. The family is told it has thirty days to get out. Family

49

in this case is a teenage girl and boy and a mother hooked up to oxygen who is chain smoking. The dead guy (husband) who showed up, summoned by them in response to the 'house eviction' notice, came home from work and promptly disappeared into the basement. This was followed shortly by a loud bang and lots of smoke. The family believes it's a boiler explosion and calls the fire department.

When you investigate deaths for a living there are a few good ways to do this. The first rule is not to be strict about the rules. It's not a case of Professor Plum and a rope, I deal with mostly natural deaths. It is my job to figure out if the death is from natural causes or not. There is no 'textbook of natural' as there is of 'unnatural' to refer to. No problem on this occasion, as there is a big hole in his chest. His upper torso, face and hands are covered in black powder residue. Actually he has two holes; one in front and another in his back which the word 'hole' doesn't quite fit anymore – it's a 'crater'. Beside the body is a rifle, but not your everyday sports store special. It's a 1862 Spencer Repeating rifle, made by the Burnside Arms Company in Hartford, Connecticut, in 1862. It's stamped on the rifle, date and all.

I know a thing or two about weapons, having personally fired most of the common killing weapons of the 20th century; some in combat. I'm holding the prototype of the modern breech-loading cartridge rifle which came out of our American Civil War and everything worse that followed. I pull back the bolt lever and out pops a large copper cartridge: empty. I searched high and low but could not find the bullet which I later found out was supposed to be a .54 caliber chunk of lead. Half of the lead was in the body; this is common in unjacketed lead rounds. This being black powder, it left an amazing amount of residue on the corpse/wound. I mostly see smokeless, jacketed, rifle bullet injuries.

I go and talk to the wife who is a cadaverous middle-aged woman, smoking Chesterfield cigarettes. I ask her for one. I'm not one of these modern medical types giving lectures about smoking. Human beings know it's bad. I also know that oxygen supports fire, but only if you're *on* fire, and smoking doesn't count. In my early days in medicine and nursing we all smoked and liked it and it was something to do in between cases. There is another reason I ask her for one; it's because the last one I had was in Vietnam twelve years before. In those days we used to get cigarettes (four) and a pack of waterproof matches in our C-ration packs, along with two chicklets (pieces of gum), six pieces of toilet paper, one packet each of coffee, sugar, powdered milk and salt and pepper for the rest of the meal. There were lots of brands of cigarettes but the most hated were Chesterfields. Towards the end of the month, when we were running low on our own brands, Chesterfields were all we had. Nothing finer at 4:30 am on watch. You get down below the sandbags and cup your hands to light one. You inhale the smoke and suck it in to get that one extra ounce of courage, while you're on the alert for something to happen that might involve you in some terminal event.

The wife tells me this story about the mortgage not being paid but she doesn't know why (and even to this day no one knows); but, sitting next to her, I kind of get the idea that being married to her is the primary reason. The husband is no blue-collar hero, but an engineer at a big engineering company. Irony of irony is that my mother worked at the same place during World War II making those famous Norden bomb-site devices, so the name of the company is familiar. My mother should have gotten a medal for her service and she is not alone, for these women worked slave hours and weeks for years.

The wife says that the rifle is a family heirloom belonging to a relative who fought in the Civil War. I don't get into the family dynamics because you don't have to be Freud to see what's going on here. The curious part is: where does he get a bullet for this 112-year-old rifle? There are no extras in the house or anything similar. No one makes this ammunition anymore and hasn't for a long time. Is it conceivable he had one bullet as an antique along with the rifle? Most likely, being an engineer, he made one; and the place he works is the kind of place he could easily make one... I'm sorry to say that I never followed up on this case. You have so many and they all seem to pile on when you want to... well. I never knew what happened to the kids but the wife was suicidally smoking herself to death. Her husband beat her to it, although *her* death certificate will say 'natural causes'.

In this next case a seventy-five-year-old man has just come home from the hospital after having a stroke which left him paralysed on one side. He had some prostate problems as well, and an in-dwelling catheter in his bladder which is driving him crazy. He cannot walk but uses a wheelchair to get around in his house, and he decides to end it all. He wheels over to a drawer in the kitchen, where he knows a 12-inch piece of rifle barrel is kept. This rifle barrel is one his young sons cut off a 22 caliber rifle about twenty years before, for reasons that our local cops know better than me. In addition to the severing cut, the barrel has half a dozen smaller cuts, for reasons unclear. He takes this barrel and wheels to his bedroom using his one good foot and hand. From a bedroom drawer, he gets a small box of .22 caliber long rifle ammunition, also very old. He also gets a pair of vice grips from a tool chest and goes into the living room. He inserts a bullet into the end of the barrel, puts the other end of the barrel into his mouth, and, holding it with his mouth, hits the base of the bullet with the flat end of the vice grips to fire the rim fire cartridge which will fire if hit hard enough – and does. The bullet exited the top of his head and hit the ceiling. That's how the family found him and how we figured it out as well.

This last case has also stuck in my mind over the years. An

elderly man, blind with diabetes, steals money from his wife's purse, little by little over several months. One day when she is out he manages to call a taxi company, which dispatches a taxi to his address after he tells them that he is blind and needs help. The location he wants is a community pavilion near the water. He's taken there and off he goes with his stick. The taxi driver was annoyed that he was paid with lots of coins, but got a nice tip. Long story short, once he's sure he's near water, he jumps and no one notices for an hour or so, until I get the call.

The thing about all three of these cases is the human ingenuity used to effect their exits. It amazes me even today. Maybe someday I'll tell you about how a guy with a technical school degree in electricity used his skills.

HOT AND COLD

I t's colder than 'a witch's tit in a brass bra', and I'm praying I don't get an outdoor case. It's tough enough in this job, but *you* should try to pronounce someone dead in a snowstorm as I have, when you have to keep brushing snow off the face and chest and the wind is howling in your stethoscope. It's not like that tonight but it's just as bad, because you have to be very careful in cold weather. All the mistaken deaths where bodies awaken in morgues happen in cold weather mostly. You shouldn't be in a hurry to say someone is dead, which is where most of the mistakes are made in my opinion. If you take your time beside a body and observe, feel, and listen, after five minutes or so you're good to go. It drives the cops crazy, but, as I told them at the beginning, I'm not checking to see if they're alive, I'm making sure they're dead, and there is a big difference: 'Dead takes longer'. Everybody (no pun) is in a hurry when it's three degrees and the wind is blowing.

We get a lot of Motor Vehicle Accidents in bad weather conditions, but cold weather finds the marginals outside freezing and somehow they wait to be found at night when I'm working. For some reason, when it gets bitter cold, I still have memories of a guy who hung himself in his living room months before, and I'm back in his freezing house where the only light is from a fish tank glowing on his decomposed face.

It also reminds me of a science fiction story I saw once. A woman is in an apartment in a city, and there is an extreme heat wave, the temps are 120 plus and the whole planet and its people are dying of heat, slowly. I think it had three suns. It turns out that the woman is hallucinating about a heatwave because she has a high fever on a planet that is icy cold. So if you think science fiction, well, you'll like this.

I had the first case. I get a call from the ER doc at our local hospital. He wants to report a case but not a death. He has an man in his eighties who has arrived in the ER with a body temperature of 57 degrees. The story is that the old guy is senile, and his family has to keep an eye on him because he tends to wander. So on this night when it's zero degrees and windy after a week of the same, they notice he is missing. They search and find him in the family pool where he has fallen through the ice. They pull him out, unconscious. Thinking he just needs to be warmed up, they put him in a bathtub to warm him up with warm water. When he doesn't wake up or start breathing they call 911 and he arrives in the ER.

Now, I started this little tale by telling you how you have to be careful pronouncing people dead in cold weather. Well, at our local hospital, the doctors are afraid of doing it (pronouncing death) so they try to warm up the body. They put the body on a respirator and a warming blanket and wait to see what happens. They do this because some children have survived fatal immersions. No adults, mind you.

While I'm talking to this ER Doc my partner comes back from a house case. He had an eighty-year-old woman who was found unconscious at home. Seems she called 911 to complain that her house was too hot and collapsed while on the phone; 911 dispatched Rescue, who transported her to a nearby hospital. The police arrived at the same time and called our office. The temperature in the house is about 110 degrees according to the thermostat. It's an old house, very dusty, and has this old-fashioned mechanical thermostat that had built up enough dust inside to short-circuit electrical connections, and the boiler had run up to a high temperature. This old woman had called 911 during the day to complain that her walls were hot, but it had been treated as a crank call. My partner said it was incredibly hot inside the house and that silverware in drawers in the kitchen was actually hot to the touch. Heat, as is well known, will drive up heart rates in anyone, but at eighty it was fatal, although no one in the ER took her temperature.

What is even more unusual is that this man's arrival in the ER is exactly the same time as this old woman's at a different hospital twenty miles away. One dead from cold and another from heat. Cases like these that we get from time to time at the morgue is when I start whistling the *Twilight Zone* theme song and looking for Rod Serling.

SUNSHINE VALLEY

I tell my partners that in the future forensic investigators will be limited to one case every other day to protect us from the mental strain. They will have recognized in a more enlightened future (perhaps) that it's cruel and unusual to expose healthcare workers to toxic levels of human contact, especially in areas of destruction, illness, and grieving family members. Those future corpse wrestlers will look back at the number of cases we handle every day and thank their good fortune they aren't living back in the bad old days that are now *my* everyday.

The name on the toe tag caught my eye more than the body itself. I was lingering in the morgue anteroom about to leave on my next case. Actually what I was doing was what most of the whole building where I work does every day – seeing what has arrived overnight. They are on stretchers in the area between the big refrigerated box where they are kept and the main autopsy room. It's not a room but a hallway, so lots of people who might not want to see or smell the new arrivals or any dead bodies, have to pass real close to those bodies to get out of or into other parts of the building. Most of the time there might be sheets protecting your sight, but, depending on what time you arrive in the stripping-off of the clothes, photographing and fingerprinting process, you will see things you will never forget. Fortunately, as long as you view these things regularly, their ability to shock or even to stay in your memory banks passes with time.

Samuel Stone was the name on the tag and it sounded familiar, a recent entry to my memory bank that was just starting to fade but enough to make me curious to see. I pulled back the sheet and it was pretty bad, but the 'USMC' 1st Marine Division tattoo said it all. I'm a 1st Marine Division vet myself although I was in the Navy not the Marines. I called over to the autopsy assistant and asked what happened and he said 'hit and run' – at 4 am across from where he lived.

The Sunshine Valley Motel. This was the wildly inappropriate name for a group of twenty single rooms that could only be described as cells, where the occupants all had life sentences and the only parole was death. I'd been there before for a routine suicide and end-stage alcoholic deaths (such deaths are as common as the Gideon bible in every drawer) and once for a tawdry homicide.

Samuel Stone was not unique; his 'Sunshine Valley' sentence was self-imposed as they all are, but he had lived a life that, in his last years, should have brought more than living in the company of men and women whose vision was limited to the bottom of vodka bottles.

I thought back two months. When I knocked, he had been

sitting in a broken chair next to a small card table, eating his evening meal of pork and beans. I could see through the curtain on the window that he had some difficulty getting up. Aided by a stout cane, he managed to rise, turn down the volume on the box with the fuzzy flickering image that passed for his television, and take two steps to the door.

I soon explained the purpose of my mission. I wondered about the last conversations, if any, with another 'Sunshine Valley' occupant, who had been found dead an hour before. His palpable pleasure at the break in his solitary routine that my visit accorded, as much as my need to learn the circumstances of his neighbor's death, kept me from leaving too quickly.

He offered me one of his cigarettes that he wasn't supposed to smoke, and a cup of coffee, the last of a meager ration until his next social security check. I threw my pack of smokes on the table and told him I'd go get us some coffee and donuts from the place across the busy highway from the motel. He was grateful and I needed a break after a long dreary day of turning corpses over to make a living.

I guess there was an unasked question on my face, because the first thing he did was start talking about how he had come to be living here. His wife had died a few years before. He lost the house to pay for her live-in health care, with a reverse mortgage. He was a retired machinist – his thickened, grease-stained fingers attested to that. He had a bad hip and needed a cane, but was happy. He had a son who was struggling under the weight of paying back his college loans, low-paying job, house, three kids and a wife who was chronically unhappy. He should have been in an adult living center but they are expensive and the VA places were filled. We talked as one old marine and one not-so-old Navy corpsman. He had been on Peleliu and been wounded after a week and his war was over. His routine now was simple and his needs were few and he seemed content with what he had. I told him to keep the smokes and thanked him for the information. 'Semper FI' was the last thing I said to him.

Driving home that day it struck me that his decision paralleled some Indian and Eskimo cultures I'd read about. In these cultures, when the elderly felt that 'their lives had been lived', they'd leave the village and live apart until death overcame them, usually due to malnutrition or exposure to the elements. This seemed to be the natural order of things, although our culture doesn't allow its members this right.

As I walked away from his body in the morgue, it occurred to me that his death might have been suicidal rather than accidental. The slowness of his gait and the darkness of the highway he had to cross had surely lent themselves to the death of a man who was waiting to die.

HAUNTED INLET

You know, spending your days with dead bodies and how they got that way can be stressful and emotional. I'm usually pretty neutral about these events now. I used to wonder why I wasn't more animated. I'm usually pretty animated otherwise. A tour in Vietnam preceded and succeeded by Emergency Room work, along with ambulance driving, Rescue Squad time and four years in general surgery, had given me enough live situations ending in terminal events to eschew any emotion.

Oh, I'm emotional, but if anything that's hated in medicine and nursing among its practitioners, it's 'emotion'. To this day I still can't say why. The job of Forensic Investigator is pretty good. You didn't see them die, so they are dead before you get there. They're not screaming, moaning, twitching, bleeding all over the place, gasping, vomiting, yelling, ashen, sweaty, cold, clammy, picking at the bedclothes, calling for family or God. They have those frightening looks on their faces as they look at you while you're trying to save them, at the same time you're telling them the lie that they are going to make it (and sometimes they do but mostly they don't).

This isn't heartlessness, just fact. The average nurse sees a thousand times more horrible things in your local hospital than any soldier in combat. Trust me, I've been in both, yet no nurse has ever been allowed the diagnosis of PTSD. You're supposed to take it and move on. So don't take offense at what I just said about the terminal events of strangers (patients). That's the professionalism they want. I never really bought into it myself, but I tried, Lord, how I tried. This morgue job has gotten to me a few times over the years and this story is about one such event.

I remember it clearly because they teach you lots of things about disease and injury but almost nothing about people or how you are going to react when, in the process of doing GOOD, something BAD happens and you have to live with it. Billy Joel says in the song *Vienna*: 'you may not know when you're right but you always know when you're wrong'. If you want to be a good doctor, you better have a real bad memory or no memory, if you want to be effective. Suffice it to say that I have all too good a memory and, when I think about my personal failures of omission and commission, it's usually at 4 am.

An old doctor told me that if you have any soul left you'll be thinking about these events and trying to rationalize them, but if not you will sleep well. So I have my soul keeping me awake some nights when I'd rather sleep, but I'm awake a lot at night with this job anyway, and I get to think about things on long dark drives. It's amazing that I spent my years from eighteen to forty-five trying to stay awake to take care of patients, and now I can't get a decent night's sleep to save my life.

I don't completely mourn it because I had the uncanny (if I may be immodest) ability to get a phone call awakening me from sleep, take the message without writing it down, and be dressed and out the door within five minutes of the call. I could go from sleep to instant action with ease. I made a lot of money in overtime with that ability. We were paid five hours overtime for each call. I'd get there so quick, I'd be home in bed sleeping for three of those five hours most nights.

So it's a spring day in a place by a inlet that for me is only filled with haunted images, as the cases I've had here are singularly brutal even by the standards of this job. They say the inlet is haunted by all who have drowned in it, and I believe it.

A recent case by a fellow investigator was a young woman from South America who was acting as a drug mule, and one of the bags ruptured and she died. The drug dealers cut her open for the stuff, then doused her with gasoline and set her on fire. Bonfires are not allowed on the shores of the inlet so, when the Fire Department arrived… surprise, surprise.

I'm at a house not too far away from the shore, where this man has blown his brains out with a shotgun. In his despondency or stupidity he has forgotten, but probably doesn't care, that his eight-year-old daughter will come home from school and find his body, and sure enough she does. You want to know what it looked like? Imagine you're eight years old and get back to me. The body is lying across a bed, with both feet on the floor, legs splayed and open at crotch level. I was so pissed off that his daughter had to see what very few people like myself and hardened detectives and my morgue wagon drivers see without puking or having nightmares for the rest of their lives, that I kicked the corpse in the balls.

At the time I had twin daughters who were the joy of my life. I would be there when they came home from school because I worked nights. They would be greeted with hugs, kisses and snacks.

To think this SOB thought so little of his own daughter still makes me mad even now. I have one wish still: that wherever this guy is – heaven, hell or in between – he still feels that kick.

HIGH SCHOOL BUDDY

'Hey, Doc! You'll like this one. He's upstairs in the bathroom. He still has the needle in his arm, just like the old days in the sixties, when I was a patrolman.' Wonderful, I hear myself say to a detective who likes me for my enthusiasm. This and the fact that he has never had any of our cases together be anything other than I said they were. He's a decent, honest, smart, detective who will never advance in our Police Department, because my partner missed a small caliber bullet wound to the back of the head of this woman with lots of hair, which was one of this detective's cases.

Today, though I can't keep the cynicism out of my voice. He's right, I'll like it, and that has me worried more than usual. I'm on overtime, because the kids want Cabbage Patch Dolls. I'd love to get that first edition of Siegfried Sassoon's poetry, and this is what has my Corpse to Sleeping Hours ratio way in favor of Corpse. WAY OVER.

I climb the stairs in a house that costs more than I'll make in five years, even with overtime. The detective pulls the sheet off the body that is seated on the commode. The head is leaning against the vanity, making a deep groove in the slack flesh of his left cheek. I pull the body upright, and I'm staring into his face when I know instantly who it is. I could use his name but even now I don't want to because I prefer to keep a different mental picture of him firmly in my mind when I think about his death and my part in it and his life.

It's September 1961 and I'm in the 9th grade in a public school after the last six years in a Catholic school. I'm not wearing a uniform. The girls sitting next to me have short skirts. They are wearing old-fashioned stockings (before pantyhose) and those skirts keep slipping up and I'm afraid to stand up most of the time.

Since O comes before S and there are no PQRs, he sat in front of me, so on that September day we became friends, or more like lord and vassal. I needed protection, and not just for sports.

I still don't know how the school managed to do it. I'm in a home room with the whole young criminal element of the two communities of which our school district was comprised in those days. If it wasn't for him I'm convinced that three things would have been certain: my nose would not be straight today, my orthodontist bill would have bankrupted my family, and I would still be paying them part of my lunch to leave me alone. I also had metal shop with these guys and they could turn out gravity knives and brass knuckles with amazing skill.

The picture I want to keep in my mind is of him turning in his seat to make some wise-guy remark or point out some rising hemline, which invariably caught his eye before mine. I was his audience and all lords need their courts, besides I was always good for test answers (*sotto voce*) and homework. He was what they then called a 'hood' (short for hoodlum), not for what he wore, although it describes the same type. As a 'hood' he had class. He had no fear of anyone or anything. This guy had more self-confidence and poise than I now possess at forty. Don't ask me about what went on in his childhood to make a boy a man before his time. That was the common denominator for all the 'hoods' I ever met. Perhaps his turning to drugs was the price you have to pay for being an adult too early. Much like the Marines I served with in Vietnam, who saw a side of the human race and themselves too early in life to believe there are any good endings.

I don't know all the facts of his life after he graduated high school. Oh yes, he graduated and he had better marks than I did. While I went to war and later college on the G.I. Bill, he avoided the war and made a pile of money in auto parts. Suffice it to say that his best years were in high school and mine were in the Navy.

If he found solace in drugs, I'm glad, because he had more than most people have now. I didn't mourn for him and don't wish he had lived longer. What makes me sad now when I think of him is that the process that made him is still considered normal in American life, and I see others like him almost every day.

WORST CASE

It was going to be one of those days which become forever imprinted on your memory, even though it was
indistinguishable from the hundred days that preceded it and
the hundred that came after it.

I awoke after a few hours sleep. I'd been out twice during
the night, the last for a nasty MVA (motor vehicle accident) at
4:15 am. A young girl, drunk, slammed her car into a pole and
was thrown to the sidewalk. Her driver's license showed her to
be very beautiful. What I saw was hard to discern as her head
had been smashed on impact with the sidewalk.

These things don't usually register for long in my psyche
as they are usually replaced every couple of hours by deaths
of other kinds. On any average day I would see three or four
corpses, not counting the ones in the morgue already, which
could be observed casually just being in the place for your
regular shift.

When I came downstairs, our two cats were licking blood
on my old Vietnam combat boots I used to wear in those days.
I got the boots out the door and hosed them down, plus the
steps to the house and the car mats, before the wife and kids
saw anything. Shit, no sleep makes you stupid. I have to pay

more attention. Damn, what can you do when you have to wade into pools of blood and motor oil to lift bodies into bags? I often have to leave all my clothes out on the porch because they are stained with blood or fluids of various kinds from corpses new and old, or when I have been in houses infested with fleas or roaches so bad that a body an hour old had a couple of hundred bites.

I spent the day with the kids. I didn't go to work in those days till 5 pm. I felt pretty good after a nice nap with the kids at 2 pm. I was still at home when I got the call, because the clerk knew I lived nearby. I didn't have to go far, about a mile or so to a really neat apartment complex of small two-storey brick buildings, filled mostly with senior citizens. I had been to this place before. I always remembered this place because I had one of my first cases there. An old man had shot himself in the head with a small .32 caliber automatic pistol. This caliber weapon is rarely seen now, everything being .38 caliber and soon to be 9mm. On his bedroom wall he had a picture from *Playboy* magazine of a young lady with her skirt awhirl. I had the same photo in my locker at work. It amazed me that this old guy and I could share the same taste in pin-ups; leg men both of us. I always think of that guy when I drive by this place.

One of the downsides of this work is the ability to remember such events, no matter where you go. It has gotten so that there is not one place in this county that I couldn't find a little patch where I had no memory of some horrific event. You know those little roadside shrines? Well, that's what I'm talking about. It was like returning to the scene of the crime. I'd roll over some chunk of ground and there it was. Deeds done in darkness, revealed in daylight by broken glass, skid marks, or disturbed earth. I could read the signs easily and have a nasty image to go with it, much to the distress of my family and friends who got used to this quirky ability of mine. I see them in my mind's eye like I see those corpses. I think that was the tag line in a recent movie: 'I see dead people.' Well, I do, on the average day, whenever I go just about anywhere.

So I arrive at the place I'm supposed to be and I speak to the cop. The body is on the second floor. It's always a bad sign when the cop is not inside the apartment. It means there is something that smells bad or is nasty to be around. The story is of an elderly woman, found dead by a neighbor, who noticed her apartment door ajar and opened it to find her dead in a chair by the door. The neighbor said she had been having real bad headaches but couldn't get an appointment with her doctor in less than two weeks.

I didn't look at the body of the woman by the door, with a towel over her face and a very strong stench of vomit. I tried looking for a light but couldn't find one. What I had was series of small lights at the top of works of art, like candles in a church. Each one illuminated a painting; all of which, to my untrained eye, looked like they belonged in a museum. In those days after Vietnam, I just had a medical education.

Long on science, short on humanities, and I had almost failed the art history course. I finally managed to pull back a heavy brocade curtain and the whole apartment was filled with a white light. The walls without art hanging on them had built-in shelves, filled with bronze and marble sculptures of great beauty and not very big in size. There were bigger works on pedestals scattered around the room. The furniture was heavy and mahogany and Victorian; that I did know from the art course. There were leather-bound books with gilt titles, and a rug with lovely colors – probably from Persia but don't quote me on that. I was in a museum. A museum this woman who was dead by the door had created for herself. The only thing missing in this apartment I thought about later was a grand piano. The bedroom was similar to the living area.

I went back to her body and removed the towel but I couldn't see her face. She is in a low-back chair with her head hanging over the back. She is fully dressed in clothes of a kind my mother wore, and her purse is beside her. Her face is not visible because it is covered with a small mountain of vomit. She had been having severe headaches for about a month or so. The autopsy revealed a ruptured aneurysm and this frequently leads to a certain kind of projectile vomiting. She had managed to make it back to her apartment before being overcome, but, in the minutes before she died, had vomited up an immense amount of vomitus onto her face. I have never seen anything like it before or since. I wiped this all off and examined the rest of her. She hadn't been dead long, maybe half a day. I really didn't want to bring her to the morgue for autopsy but that doctor of hers was away and the covering doctor wouldn't sign the death certificate despite the fact that I told him everything was OK.

So when people who find out what I do for a living, at parties or in casual conversations, invariably ask me for the worst case I have ever had, I tell them this story. They always seem disappointed. I don't know why. I have seen a lot of terrible things, but to see this woman who created this temple of beauty and refinement and then became the ugly, smelly, thing in it – well, for me, this is my worst case, because I've seen cats licking blood off of my boots and seen old men with bullet holes in their heads who like the same pin ups I do. DISAPPOINTED?

GILDED SHORES

I hate these cases. It's not the cases, it's the having to drive an hour or so to get there if I'm lucky (longer if I'm not), for ten minutes work. I shouldn't complain, I know. I've had some interesting cases in the playground of the rich and famous. I have mostly locals and poor, but I've had some minor characters in rich houses filled with books and art and someday I think... well.

I had a lovely quiet afternoon once with a nurse I liked very much out there. I was on overtime, so I took her along to a hanging. She waited in the car while I did what I do. We stopped and had lunch in an expensive restaurant and sat near someone famous, window-shopped, and death left me alone for once. He was not that far away, as this nurse was in the early stages of a nasty disease called scleroderma. I liked her, she was sweet, great nurse; hope it was quick.

The last interesting case I had out there was the Cyclops. He was not really a Cyclops. He was a big guy, a retired grounds keeper on an estate, who had squamous cell cancer of the nose from his years in the sun. It had eaten a hole in his face that had taken both eyes. I say Cyclops because, as a kid, I a saw a movie with Kirk Douglas as Ulysses. The Cyclops eats some crew members and Kirk puts his one eye out. It looked a lot like this guy in death. Forgive me, mister, but I didn't sleep for weeks after seeing that movie as a kid and, well… FORGIVE ME..

Fortunately, in this case, I got the call at a little after 5 pm. The big wave of traffic hits our county about 6 pm, so I was ahead of the rush. I can really speed for most of the way and highway patrol will give me a break as I'm doing 85 and they are looking for guys above this. I know how to stay behind the leader who's doing more, but I've been nailed by them. Usually the badge works, but not with all. The first time I got a ticket, we had an old Buick with a 400 hp engine and set up for high speed pursuit, given to us by, of all people, the highway patrol. The Health Department was too cheap to give us cars in those days.

The other thing about shores' cases is that you're out of position, way out to respond to anything else. Almost always, you're half way out and you get two other cases at the opposite end of the county, so instead of being one hour late, you're two or three.

The case today is another of the typical stories from families. Tried to reach the dead guy all week, but at least they didn't wait till 10 pm. This case is on the other side of the shores in Poole. It's only a marginally shorter drive. I used to duck hunt in a lovely cove across from a convent there for retired nuns.

This man is dead on the kitchen floor and looks like he's

been a week dead. He's none too ripe and has a disinviting viscid greasy pool surrounding him which I have to wade into. He's a skinny man who hasn't been eating much but has been drinking a lot. He likes scotch and the label is one I haven't seen in a long time – 100 Pipers (bagpipers). I didn't think they made it anymore. I had a friend in the Navy, who at his going-away party drank thirty-five scotch and waters, 100 Pipers. The only place he went after was to the hospital for three days. We all put him there by buying him drinks.

I pulled the body up into a sitting position by both arms and he looked different. Then I saw that his scalp was still stuck to the floor. It's not tissue but a full wig which is perfectly in shape. It's an Elvis wig with the big DA (duck's ass) front. It looks funny on the floor. The detective and I have a laugh. He was a good singer and had some good songs, but what I hate now about Elvis is that everyone in America wants to imitate him or they say how much he meant to them and how he's inspired their lives. Give me a break!! Turns out this guy is seventy. Amazing. We bag the guy and I start the long drive back.

It's a funny thing about wigs and hair in men. I've been bald since my late twenties and, when I look in the mirror, it always seems there is a different guy than the one who is supposed to be looking back at me. The guy with hair. I'd always say to the kids, that if I get rich I'd get a hair piece like Sean Connery or Frank Sinatra. I'll never be that rich, I'm sure.

I'm thinking about all this when I remember a weird event

from my early days, when I worked for a six-man multi-specialist surgical group. I was a new graduate and my boss was the chief of surgery at this community hospital. My arrival was not particularly welcomed by the other attending MDs and especially the nurses, being one of the new Physician Assistant profession – although no one reacted with more venom than the chief of Radiology – I was like a red flag to a bull to him. I didn't know this and I started off by thinking I could ask him a question. Forget about it, he even questioned my right to look at his X-rays. I asked my boss to intervene and he did, but it didn't help much. He was nasty whenever he could be when I was around. I was around the X-ray department a lot because we had a lot of patients, plus there was a lovely young divorced file clerk making eyes at me and I was definitely making them back.

This radiologist was pretty nasty to just about everybody else as well. He was an imposing guy, tall and thin – about 6 feet 4 inches – and completely bald. We always thought that being exposed to all that X-ray was how he had lost his hair, but he had a medical condition called Alopecia Totalis. He had been bald since adolescence and he was in his mid-fifties when I knew him.

So, imagine the shock when one day in he walks with a full head of blond hair, and I mean full. This was mid 1970s. Even more than his appearance was that his personality had completely changed as well. It's as if a light had been switched on with this wig, and his negative personality had become friendly and positive. It was like Scrooge on Christmas morning. He smiled, laughed, was joyful, mirthful, and patient. I don't think he uttered an impatient word after. He never apologized for his previous behavior. After a while, it was so nice to be in his company that myself and others never held his former self against him. No one that I know of ever remarked to him about his hair or his reasons for the wig. You have to understand what hospitals are or were then. Little closed communities of people, with the big MDs and small floor sweepers all wanting to be part of something good, decent, taking care of people, your neighbors, your families and friends. The shock was not his hair but the personality change, welcomed like a lost friend or relative, and it made the staff happy the way that the wig made him happy. In a million years you would have never thought it possible that this man in particular would do this, which made our joy even greater. I know it sounds like I'm going way overboard – and maybe I am, because I was given special consideration, given our history. He taught me a lot about reading X-rays and radiology, which was never my strong point. That lovely divorced file clerk taught me a few things as well, mostly anatomy. Hers.

I had a chest X-ray in this old hospital recently, as my doctor lives nearby. There is a plaque in the new radiology department to this man's memory. I ask the young X-ray tech if she knew him. She didn't. I tell her he was the nicest doctor I ever met.

FAMILY PLACE

Jesus Christ on a crutch. I hate rush-hour cases in this county. It's like being a salmon swimming upstream against three dams, a few grizzly bears and some scumbag in LL Bean waders with a fishing pole that costs more than a village in Central America trying to take you home to stuff, just to get to the scene of these accidents.

Fortunately, after all the years of chasing corpses at all hours of the day and night in this county, I know how to get there quicker by taking a major road through an industrial park. Unfortunately, it's on a nasty strip of highway with five major cemeteries along it. I say unfortunately, not only for the victims but for me. This accident is across from the cemetery where all my family are buried. I have been on this road before for accidents, and it really gets to me to be pulling corpses into body bags in site of where your parents and grandparents are buried.

This MVA is pretty nasty, with multiple cars and victims. It's a four-lane highway running north and south. Whatever the speed limit is, no one follows it. It's on the borderline between two precincts with minimum coverage. People speed here because of all the cemeteries. Who wants to go slow past a graveyard, especially at night? I once had a case where this cemetery was selling to local contractors the excess soil that accumulates with burials. The coffin takes up the space and after X number of burials you have a pretty good size pile of dirt. They sell this 'spoil', as it's called, to local contractors for lots of uses. The contractor in the case I was involved in had built a house on a wet piece of ground and had to build up the soil, so he got a couple of truckloads of this spoil, and then put topsoil on top of it. The new owners unfortunately had a labrador retriever who dug a hole in this new lawn and dragged into the house the severed leg of a person who had had surgery – the leg was covered in bandages. I think one person in this cemetery is one leg short some time soon.

These cemeteries are opposite a huge cemetery where my folks are buried. A little north of these cemeteries is a big cemetery whose name ends in 'Lawn', and then the huge Veterans Administration cemetery where my uncle Jack Moran is buried; my mother's brother. He was a Sergeant in D company 502nd regiment of 101st Airborne, who got a bronze star and a purple heart at Bastogne and who is buried near the front gate. It opened in 1951 and he died in 1952, seven years after World War II. He was thirty-five. As Raymond Chandler, the famous novelist, said of his World War I experience as sergeant of a platoon in the Canadian army that was wiped out, 'Once you go over the top into the face of a machine gun, life is never the same'. I still have my uncle Jack's overseas foot locker with his stencil on it. My uncle Jack and I share a first name and an Irish heritage, and we both know what Chandler was talking about, all too well. I never met my uncle. I was five years old when he died so we never got to talk about war.

I went to Bastogne a few years back. I saw where he fought. The woods have all grown back but the locals are still pulling bombs and occasional corpses out of them every year since. I stood in front of a building dedicated to the men of the 502nd and scooped up a few handfuls of dirt and put it in a plastic bag. I brought it back and placed it in front of his grave along with a couple of tulips. The VA hates planted flowers on graves, and some squirrels ate the bulbs, but that soil is still there and it makes me glad when I think of him. I know the thing about this accident location that breaks my heart is that it is where I have one of my dearest childhood memories.

I can remember it with that clarity which only advancing years brings. It's 1958 or '59 and I'm with my father in this cemetery, which in those days seemed so far away and a long drive from our house. My father is crying like a baby, something I have never seen and I remember it to this day much as the way he wept when I got on a train to go to Vietnam. Now he's not too far away from his mother, his brother and his brother's wife (who we all miss as the great Italian cook, since we all married non-Italian wives) and I weep at his grave as he did so long ago. For my mother as well.

This cemetery is famous/infamous at our office. It's a

curious aspect of a medical examiner's life that you get grief-stricken family members who actually kill themselves on the graves of their dead loved ones. This particular cemetery has had a greater percentage of these cases than usual. The reason I think is because there is a famous/infamous gun shop about a quarter of a mile away. It's in a strip mall of a major highway, that somehow really defines what I have grown to hate and I wish a vicious death for all who have made it so. This gun shop is known for the bumper stickers it gives away free: 'Make love not war but be prepared for both'; 'They will get this gun when they pry it from my cold dead fingers'.

The last makes me laugh as I have literally done that – 'prying guns out of their cold dead fingers' – not in defense of second amendment rights murdered by gun control advocates but from those who have died by their own hands.

We used to have a standing joke at retirement parties. When the person who had pulled the pin (ie. retired to the hand grenade that retirement life could be) was a hunter of any sort, they would get an expensive rifle or shotgun which we would all contribute to pay for, and the joke on its presentation was that it had only been used once.

The good thing from an investigative point of view about these gun shop suicides was the receipt. You'd find the guy dead, next to the box on top of the grave, and the receipt was inside. It went something like this.

```
10/19/1987 2:02 pm
Shotgun pistol grip   $79.99
1 box shells 12 ga    $15.99
Tax                   $ 3.59
Total                 $99.57
```

As an investigator you really have to like guys like this, because I pronounced him dead on 10/19/1987 at 3:27 pm. Just about long enough to stroll over from the gun shop, load the gun with one shell, say a prayer and do the deed. Then for someone to hear the shot, investigate and call the police. Case closed and on to the next. NO complications – which is big if you're a detective or forensic investigator.

I have other memories of this area adjacent to the graveyard. I had a guy who was hit by a car speeding by the graveyard, late at night. He was one of those central American immigrants who have invaded our county in recent years, thanks to Ronald Reagan's policies which have destroyed their countries so they come to the USA. He had a face that looked like it belonged on a Mayan temple, and green feet. He had been living in the wooded areas adjacent to the cemeteries some place, and his feet were wet and green from the dye from his cheap sneakers. He might have been an agricultural worker, as so many of these men are. We buried him in a pauper's grave, and never got an ID.

It all reminds me of Lyndon Johnson's war which I

participated in. In those days it was all about South Vietnam and its corrupt government which we supported.

I think of all this as I sit under a tree, after I have officially pronounced the four corpses dead. That's all the cops want. I now have to wait as they videotape the scene, after all the photographs, before we can remove the bodies. I see all these ghosts but they no longer scare me. This is life. My life. I'm alive.

> *'Happy the man and happy he alone*
> *who can call today his own.*
> *He who secure within can say*
> *Tomorrow do thy worst*
> *because I have lived today…'*

John Dryden (1631–1700)

VETERANS DAY

There is a character in the Erich Maria Remarque novel *Three Comrades* called Valentin Hauser. The novel is about German veterans re-adjusting to life after World War I. The storyline about Valentin Hauser is that he has devoted his life completely to celebrating having survived the war. The rest of the characters are trying to forget about the war. Valentin remembers every hour, day, week, month of the war. Nothing is as important in the life he survived to live than enjoying every hour, day, week, month, forever after.

This character describes my life completely after Vietnam. Like him, I remember every hour and day of the eleven months I served in Quang Nam province. I knew it was a bad place to be but it turns out 85 percent of all Marine Corps casualties dead and wounded during the seven years the Corps was there occurred in old Quang Nam.

Imagine you could be born as an adult and get to re-live your life all over again. Then you have some idea, if you have imagination, of what it felt like for me to have come home alive.

If there is a howling blizzard and I have to go out in it to pronounce somebody dead at home, I think this is so much better than humping a pack in 120-degree heat. If it's pouring rain and I sit at my window, dry, looking out, I can remember monsoon days damp, wet and cold and the thundering roar of torrential rain on the tin roof of our hooch. If it's hot and I have a cool drink of water, I remember the hot (chlorine-treated) terrible-tasting water we had to drink so much of it made you thirstier. If I'm hungry I can cook up some pasta and not eat out of cans: beans and meatballs and ham and lima beans (ham and MFs to Marines). So if you add in a shower every day, underwear, flush toilets with real toilet paper, clean clothes, fresh vegetables, meat, bread, whiskey and sex – well, Jimmy Stewart doesn't have a clue as to what a wonderful life is. All this, plus – and it's a big one – people not trying to kill you and being able to walk just about anywhere without looking where you put every footstep, knowing there is a good chance you'll wind up like what was left of the guy you put in a bag a few weeks earlier after he stepped on a 155m artillery shell booby trap. There is one other thing I liked about Valentin and this book, and that is it's about soldiers who have lost their war. After Vietnam there wasn't much insight into what losing feels like.

It's Veterans Day when, if anything all, my enjoyment of being alive is even stronger. I always try to work on Veterans Day (Armistice Day) and Memorial Day (Decoration Day). I like to call these days by their old names. The meaning was truer in the days before the Department of War became the Defense Department. We haven't had a war since the last declared Congressional war, World War II. It's the last time we won as well. These undeclared Defense Department wars have been illegal and we have lost every one. Working gets me out of having to attend any Veterans Day remembrances in my neighborhood. It's mostly the World War II and Korean guys marching. There are three Vietnam vets in my neighborhood – me, a guy who has a Silver Star and a sailor who served on a ship. The rest, draft dodgers all. Since I remember every day and month, I don't feel I'm slighting those who died by not going. Besides, all this honoring just leads to more dead to honor.

I remember marching in all those parades as a kid after World War II and recall that it's partly how I wound up in Vietnam, which I survived. Memorials just point out the sacrifice, not the peace it brought, and keeping that peace is a better memorial to their sacrifice than making more soldiers, bullets and bombs, where most of the American budget goes. My fellow investigators are glad to let me work the day. I'm the only Vietnam veteran in our office.

My faithful post-war guide Robert J. Lifton MD says, in *Home from the War*, that this is a common view of veterans even as far back as ancient Greece. We have been allowed to kill. As grateful as non-veterans are that we did this, they harbor fear of us. I used to wear my Vietnam combat boots and a Marine Corps dress greatcoat in winter when I first started working as an investigator, but the boots fell apart and I got too fat for the coat. Most times on Veterans Day, I would get a veteran who would kill himself.

Today's case is early in the morning and not too far from my house. It's on the poor side of town. Usually I get the vet suicides later in the day after heavy drinking. This guy is a Vietnam vet with a gunshot wound to the head. He is a few years younger than me, a Marine, seated in a VW, bright orange in color, in the street in front of his house. The rifle he put in his mouth has caused an explosion of his head, which has left virtually nothing above the neck. The windows of this orange VW are red with blood and brains so you can't see anything inside. There is a big hole in the roof where the bullet exited. I go and talk with his wife and family friends. I tell them I'm a vet. Some of his Marine friends are there and after I tell them what unit I was with, they are glad to know a Nam doc is in control and will give the family the truth. I get a better history of this fellow's trouble from his Marine buddies than his wife. It seems that this guy is one of these PTSD fellows who just can't shake his war experience.

It's one of those ironic episodes with which most lives are filled that, having hated high school and barely graduated, I joined the Navy in the last months before graduation. With me thinking I was finally free of sitting in a classroom, the Navy sent me to school for the next year. I graduated a Navy Corpsman specializing in neuro-psychiatric problems. I had applied for the psych school because my girlfriend was nearby at a local college and I was desperate to be near her, rather than for any love of psychiatry, and ironically two months into the school she left me. So here I was in the middle of the war working the male enlisted psychiatric wards as well as officers, female military and civilian, plus neurology. Twelve days on, two off. Port and starboard they called it. Two of those twelve were fourteen-hour days at the National Naval Medical Centre, Bethesda, Maryland

Well, you would think I'm going to tell of the shell-shocked Vietnam vets I saw, but you'd be wrong. I had only one from February 1966 to May 1968. We had mostly stateside screw-ups, legitimate recruits with mental illness whom the Navy let in because the recruiting standards were so low. Remember, there was a draft so you had to go. We had a recruit from India who, after arriving, got a draft notice and decided to join the Navy instead. He was a problem from the beginning but we got him after he was found confused and wandering after trying to shoot the commander of his base with a bow and arrow.

We had some great psychiatrists. Each chart had a narrative summary and ended with a diagnosis. One doctor wrote of a manipulative female Marine: 'petulance is her mode, promiscuity is her manner'. Another psychiatrist was a small German fellow who had a broad German accent for a Navy doctor. He was never without some form of tobacco product in his mouth – pipe, cigar, cigarette. He was also always fondling a huge fountain pen and had a great signature. Freud had the same problem with tobacco. Working on the women's ward was tough as some dopey corpsman invariably would have sexual relations with the females and find themselves transferred to the Aleutian Islands, if they were lucky, or worse, the 9th Marines – 'The Walking Dead'.

The CO was a patrician Boston Brahmin who had pioneered the modern treatment of 'combat fatigue', as it was called after World War II and Korea. They were treated close to the front with a hot shower, clean clothes, a good meal and sedation for forty-eight hours, and 95 percent were anxious to return to their units within five days or a week at most. Never, in all the time I was in Psychiatry at Bethesda, did anyone notice anything that latterly became PTSD, myself included. We had about two dozen psychiatrists and a whole big Psychology Department. Nothing... Nada... Zippo... Zilch... Zero.

You would think these smart doctors would have seen something and maybe they did after I left. I spent every year after war in medicine at some level and it wasn't till the late '70s, after the soldiers and marines had been home for years and began to self-destruct, that it was recognized, or at least some definition of symptoms came about.

So what is PTSD? I think PTSD is just war guilt.

There is a funny reaction to having been in a war and then coming home. Things you did there, that seemed so natural, take on an ominous aspect viewed at home. Remember what

I said about being allowed to kill? All of a sudden at the family dinner table on Sunday, usually after church, you think 'Oh my God, I've killed'. Lots of guys start to freak out at what they have done in the name of defending their country. Want to know why 'Cool Hand Luke' is cutting heads off of parking meters to get arrested? Well, he's done something he's not proud of in World War II (like shooting civilians) and it haunts him. They cut that out of the movie. Ruins recruiting, you know, in 1966.

I think this guy in the VW is one of them. This fellow has done something he can't live with now that he's back in the land of the free. I knew a vet who had a drinking problem and was fired from just about every job he had. He progressed to be a full-time drunk who I would see from time to time. He finally told me he had shot a kid in Vietnam accidentally.

The Marines I was with on a small hill outside Danang, had recently been attacked by an NVA sapper squad. Consequently, everyone was on high alert especially as the sun started to set. There was a problem with the villagers trying to sneak into the nearby dump to scrounge things to sell or give to local VC. It was mostly kids who were kept away by random potshots. There was a small guard in the dump during the day but they would leave around sunset and, in the brief period before it got too dark, the nearby village kids and some adults would begin to get close to the dump, which wasn't fenced. They only had a limited time to get in or out because once it got dark we'd shoot at anything that moved.

Our hill was 60 meters high. From this height we had two 106 recoilless rifles, which we fired on suspected enemy mortar or rocket sites we could see firing on Danang. The back side of the hill gave us a view of the dump border and the kids. At first it was just a random pot-shot, far from anyone, into the sand, but as the kids got bolder, sensing we wouldn't actually shoot them, they would get closer to the dump. It didn't seem at the time as bad as it sounds now to tell it, as those bullets were pretty far from hitting anyone, until one evening when a seventeen-year-old Marine hit a kid. Fortunately, the kid was not seriously injured. The Marine Corps investigated. The family got 35 dollars and the Marine was fined. A week later, the two guards in the dump were killed when a booby trap put in a pile of tin cans exploded next to a small awning, there to protect them from the sun. The seventeen-year-old Marine who shot the kid was killed four months later by another seventeen-year-old Marine who was handling his M16 carelessly, and this Marine was killed accidentally by another Marine.

I was the only medical person around and although I wanted to go to this kid's aid after he was shot we had already set up our trip flares and booby traps and the kid was carried off to the nearby ville. I also held a little clinic every day at the base of the hill for the kids who all had these terrible sores on their legs mostly. I'd put on Furacin crème and wrap them up and they would pull them off later. I had to treat a young girl with a septic finger and I managed to give her a penicillian shot. It cured her finger and the sores on her legs at the same time. Turns out these sores are a disease called 'Yaws' and pencillin works great. So I cured the whole ville of this disease.

So now I spend my days happy to have survived, and put veterans in body bags to make a living, but I don't have PTSD and I'm not alone. Not one of the corpsmen I knew in the Psychiatric Department at Bethesda, who later went to Vietnam like me, has it.

I'm convinced that if the dead could come back to life, they wouldn't waste it by whining about things they saw. We were all volunteers in the Navy and Marines, so you have no one to blame for being there. If nothing else, take your private grief and turn it into something better that benefits the human race. Don't waste the life you lived to survive; it makes a mockery of those who died. You didn't suffer as much as they did, Gyrene.

When I was in surgery we got a student who said he'd been in Vietnam with the Marines. I tried to help him out, but he was a screw-up and my bosses gave him a bad mark. Years later he became a recognized expert and proponent of the new PTSD theory (having, he said, been a combat vet) and pioneered the care of PTSD vets. I thought that it was nice to see him move on and do well. I liked him and maybe surgery wasn't his thing. So imagine my surprise when I meet him at a medical conference twenty years later and in casual conversation about our Navy years I came to realize from the things he was saying that he'd never been in Vietnam. He had been a corpsman, but not a Marine corpsman.

In recent years I've come across two corpsmen I served with in the Navy – one at Bethesda who didn't go to Vietnam but to a hospital ship, and the other I knew in Vietnam – both 100 percent disabled from PTSD.

Besides, Kipling knows the real reason for most post-war angst:

> *We have done with hope and honor*
> *We are lost to love and truth*
> *We are dropping down the ladder*
> *Rung by rung*
> *And the measure of our torment*
> *Is the measure of our youth*
> *God help us we knew the worst too young.*

BLACK BANKS

It's a bitter cold day in January. We hardly get these kind of days any more. The creek is roiling with small waves in the inlet where I have my decoys set out for broadbill duck in a classic 'J' pattern. It's about 10 degrees and, with the wind, a lot colder. I couldn't be happier, as for almost forty years I have been hunting ducks. I am an old man now, but I remember when I was young when it really was cold. The winter of 1976 always stands out as a benchmark but in the early '60s it was so cold that the salt water creeks froze and you could walk across them. So, like an old Indian, I've lived fifty-six winters and I know a thing or two about life and hardship.

I'm freezing as only a man who smoked too many cigarettes as a young man has his feet telling him. I don't smoke any more. Despite this, duck hunting has never been as much fun as in the days when a thermos of coffee and a pack of Marlboro were my only breakfast. A 'soldier's breakfast', as they say about soldiers, but I guess being in Vietnam with the Marines counts.

On moonlit December morns at 5 am I'd skim across the bay and leave phosphorescent wakes with my small duck boat and settle in, after setting decoys, and enjoy lovely sunrises and sunsets. In those days I would be out all day. I have been doing this since I was sixteen but now it always reminds me a little of what Vietnam was like, where I'd be on watch from 4 am to sunrise, with an M-16 and a few grenades and watch the dawn progress from black to gray to white.

It's a slow day, mostly mergansers and the occasional buffle-head. I really don't care that much about killing ducks any more and I think it's about time I stopped doing this, after all the death I've seen and I see every day. Now it's mostly doing things I did as a young man to prove I'm not old. I always enjoyed the beauty of the sky and sun, but now even more I enjoy just being out here on the lonely marshes where I was a boy and remarkably they are as devoid of people now as then. I know it may sound fanciful but it's the only part of my life that has any continuity with that of a sixteen-year-old boy. I'm an educated man now and have lots of responsibilities, but when I'm in this boat and in this creek – well, let's just say I'm where I should be, and some day when I die I want to have my ashes spread here.

As I said, it's a slow day and my feet are freezing more than usual. I get in the decoys with some difficulty and the front of the boat has an ice-cap on it that holds the nose down, but these Barnagatt Bay sneak boxes are more stable with ice on the front. I head home with wind and spray covering the boat. I've driven home in worse, and with game wardens chasing me 'cause I was dusking (shooting after dark). My boat was so shallow-bottomed I could go through Beggi's Creek and be home before these guys could feel my warm motor hood.

As I pull up to the dock, I see my father. I say 'Pop, what are you doing here?' He has tears in his eyes and he says that it was so bad (weather-wise) he was afraid for me and came to see I got back okay. I said 'Pop! I like it when it's like this!' but he doesn't seem to understand. Then I understand that he's old now, almost seventy-eight years old, and in his mind I'm still that sixteen-year-old boy. He's been frightened for me maybe as much as when I was younger and his anxiety has driven him to come and see that I'm safe. I'm overwhelmed with his concern and walk him back to his car. He lives two minutes from where I keep my boat. I tell him I'll stop by as soon as I have cleaned up the boat. As he drives away, I think about two things.

It's 1968 and I have been in the Navy for three years, but now I have orders for Vietnam and we have fooled my mother into thinking I'm just going to Okinawa. He knows that's not true, so we are at the train station and we go to a nearby bar (something that never happened ever, before or after). I try to tell him that there's a possibility that I won't be coming back (I didn't really want to believe it myself) and, since we had never had a conversation about anything (that's the way men were back then) – well, we just didn't get to the point, as much as I wanted to tell him. The tears in his eyes when I left told me he knew; and mine weren't dry. I came back and no one was happier for me than him, 'cause my mother made his life miserable, blaming him for my being in Vietnam. See, he was a

Navy Air Reservist and every month he'd go to a Navy base in uniform and for two weeks a year he would be on active duty at Guantanamo or Jacksonville, Florida.

In November 1968, I was wounded in the arm by shrapnel from our own exploding munitions and admitted to NSA Danang. I begged them not to notify my parents (very small wound). Yet one Sunday a few days later a Navy officer showed up on the doorstep of our house; my mother never recovered from the shock of the seconds it took my parents to realize he was not there to tell them I was dead, but just wounded. In November 1968 I'd just been in Vietnam for four months and had seven more to go.

The second thing is that in June 1961, when I was fourteen years old and just graduated from Catholic School, on the last Saturday my father said he had gotten me a job for the summer at a boatyard. I was so naïve that my whole family having breakfast didn't clue me in. After eating we all got into his car and drove to a Marine boat yard close to where we lived. The man who owned the place, was supposed to be there when we arrived, but he wasn't, so a lovely man named Mr Frank acted as the owner. My father spoke to him and I was told to get some boat cushions from a nearby locker and take them down to a boat at the dock. Imagine my surprise when, approaching this boat, there was a sign in the cockpit that said 'Happy Birthday/Graduation!' A 16-foot speedboat with a 35 hp Evinrude engine.

I'm standing on the same dock at the same place with the same man who worked his ass off to buy his son (probably with the overtime money he made with the big snowstorm of 1961) this boat when I was fourteen. He is still worried about me and we are both old men.

What can you say to such a man? Nothing. Just weep that he is no longer in the world to worry about you.

THE BAD SEED

It's one of those bright sunny days bursting with life and, still being a youngish man, I respond to the joy of being alive while I drive to my next case. I think one of the reasons I stay in this job is that I'm not trapped in an office or hospital but free to travel about on sunny days like this.

Emily Dickinson said it best: 'I feel like a funeral in my brain', so in the midst of the joy it's always at the expense of, or heightened by, the other. I can't define it any better so I let Emily speak for me. She is not alone. With most of the things I experience, I use someone else's words to explain the emotions I feel. Undertakers use the same old tired phrases as doctors and have to use them even when they might feel different because there really aren't many ways in English to talk about death and the feelings that go with it. I just got into the habit because I was sick of hearing and thinking the same old things. I'm insightful but had no language, so now I use the phrases and insights of people who have commented better on the human heart or condition and said things I couldn't or never would say. I have a small book filled with quotes and aphorisms, ideas and words by the great and the small that I have gleaned from my wide reading. I'm a referential man.

I like to think that this line of work is so unique that I am exploring a completely new field. Who else spends his days with three or four corpses and their histories and lives and how they became corpses? It's history, medicine, science, narrative, literature, and from all this I make choices and come to conclusions. I really have almost complete freedom of action within my sphere. I'm so free it's scary, but you will never know finer work in life – paid work, that is.

This all reminds me very much of how modern psychiatry was created. The mentally ill were generally under care of Neurology at the turn of the century in Vienna. Neurologists had plenty of work with the mentally ill as there was very minimal neurosurgery in those days. The psychotic have always been institutionalized but everyone else, even if their families had money, was basically disregarded by neurology because they didn't know how to make them better.

Freud, who has trained as a neurologist, can't get work because he is Jewish and he can't get a break from the doctors in Vienna who could send him patients. If you're a specialist you need feeders (GPs) to send their patients to you. Freud is desperate and a fellow neurologist tells him about the mentally ill daughters and wives of rich men in Vienna whom he has seen and had some limited success in treating. The rest, as they say, is history. So perhaps this is why I feel as I do.

There is another Freud connection. Freud didn't know how to classify or figure out the things he was seeing and feeling and thinking about so he had to fall back on ancient Greek for the Oedipus complex and societal, mythic and totemic symbols. So I use Emily Dickinson, Dashiell Hammett, Herman Hesse, Ivan Illich, George Carlin and Randy Newman among others

This has been a rather long preamble to the following tale.

One day, out in a lovely place, wooded, quiet and peaceful, due to the fact that it's in a rather exclusive part of the county and only the very wealthy reside where people have been living for 400 years. The woods have been chopped down and grown back two or three times, a Labrador retriever, being true to its nature, brings home a rather large bone. Its owner, on seeing it, thinks it's possibly human but disregards this idea (a number of times as it turns out), but by the end of the week this dog has brought home a number of bones, now including a human jaw bone, and the owner calls the police.

The police have their own dog that follows the retriever's scent out to the wooded area about a mile away and finds the rest of the skeleton under a tree, which has a noose hanging from a limb above the body. The skeleton turned out to be that of a nineteen-year-old boy whose family lived adjacent to a large estate whose secluded grounds and decaying mansion (a Gatsby palace if ever there was one) were familiar to me before someone burned it down smoking dope in the late '70s.

Dental records officially identified the young man and the death certificate listed suicide as manner of death. This was four years before I started work as an investigator. We had a young forensic pathologist who was rummaging around in the main cooler and had found the remains of this young man still unclaimed. He wanted the bones as his private exemplar. He wanted me to get permission from the family. I drafted a letter and sent it, explaining what he wanted, along with a consent form. I got no reply, so I sent it again, registered, and again got no reply. After about six weeks this pathologist was bugging me to go to the residence and speak to the family, so one evening I arrived at their door.

It was a large, well-furnished house, and the young man's father and I spoke in his book-lined den. He had gotten the two letters but he hoped we would forget about it so hadn't replied. He quickly signed the consent form and didn't ask what the bones would be used for. I was about to leave, but I guess the weight of the look on my face got to him, and he began to explain why he was doing it. He said he had four children, all about two or three years apart, three sons and a daughter. All the rest had been, and still were, model young adults and were leading productive, important and interesting lives in their chosen professions. This one son was completely different and had been a problem from day one. He was always in fights, got poor grades, was caught stealing and, as he got older, in the late '60s, started using drugs. He had run away on a few occasions, usually to return after a few weeks. When he disappeared the last time, they waited a few weeks before filing a missing persons report. It was three years later that his body was found by the dog. He felt that somehow this child was not his child, being completely different from its siblings, even though they had all been raised with the same loving care. Something he still couldn't understand, all these years later. I thanked him for telling me. The young pathologist left shortly after and didn't take the bones with him. I'm not sure where they wound up, but we had lots of bones, that's for sure, with no names or families who might have wanted them back if they knew where they were.

The thing that bothered me at the time, since I had no children myself, was that the father didn't want the bones. He could have buried them in a grave somewhere, with or without a stone. We do that for John Does. There was not one bond of love or concern here. Strange, the ways of HUMANS, I thought, but I was young and quite naïve in some ways about them: HUMANS.

About six years later I got a call, one Monday afternoon of a three-day holiday weekend, to an apartment complex. It's one of these real anonymous places that, along with trailer parks, especially fill what's left of my soul with the kind of high-grade fear – much like when in Vietnam, having completed a road sweep looking for mines, I had to get in a Jeep to drive back to base over the road we just swept. I see my future perhaps in these places.

The apartment complex is about twenty-five years old, but Stephen King writes about places like this. It has the concentrated essences of all the dead hopes and desires of its occupants, and they know it and I feel it.

Fading paint, dead bushes and shrubbery, rust, stinks, rotten wood, grey halls with no lights, dirty windows that don't open, many broken and taped-up, leaves in the gutters, broken damaged doorways and replaced locks and dead bolts, mangy cats with visible scabs, and dogs so overfed and barely exercised that they hobble to shit in a parking lot that is filled with holes and weeds and no car less than ten years old and dirty.

The cop tells me the parents found their son dead in his bedroom and called police, no ambulance. They are seated on a couch in the living room of a small two-bedroom apartment. I say hello and tell them that I will examine their son first and come back to talk to them. He's a thin young man in his early twenties, face down in bed. His face is deeply discolored purple by non-blanching dependent lividity and he's still in rigor mortis, which breaks with moderate pressure. This indicates he's been dead at least a day or two, but then I notice a faint greenish discoloration to the lower abdomen, which puts it closer to three days. I systematically search his room (forensic investigators can do this without a warrant in suspected non-criminal cases) and find some pills in his pants pocket and marijuana in a desk drawer. There are no marks of violence or injury. I tell the cop to call Crime Scene to come and photograph the body. I call the detectives and tell them I have an overdose death and they will come and investigate as well.

I speak with the parents, although the father does all the talking. They say he came home late Friday night and has been in his room ever since. Their son has a history of drug abuse and a low-paying job and still lives at home. The parents have been home all weekend as well, yet did not enter the room or call him till late this afternoon. They look at me; I look at them as they tell me this. The wife continues to say nothing and the father says they didn't know how to stop him using drugs and they pretty well have left him alone all the time to come and go as he pleased.

I tell them I don't know what he died from, that I have found some drugs and that an autopsy will be performed. They never asked how long he had been dead and I didn't say. When the detectives arrive I tell them this story and leave. Their report says the parents never entered his room. The cause of death was drugs and alcohol. This boy was their only child and they didn't check on him for three days. How could they sit there for that time and what are they thinking, now that they have found him dead, about having waited? Now you know why I hate these places.

You would think, having witnessed these two previous events, I'd be prepared for the third and you would be wrong.

This is the real debilitating thing about this business – that, after a while, when you have seen the most horrible, disgusting, obscene, tragic, sad, miserable things that can be seen on this planet, there is always something worse waiting around the corner and you know what? 'I CAN'T WAIT TO SEE IT.'

In fact everything before has given you a badass attitude that says, 'I CAN SEE ANYTHING', and sadly it comes true.

So one evening a few years later, shortly after I get to work, I get a call to a neighborhood where life is more up-scale than its neighboring towns.

It had been a long winter with many severe snow squalls and it was still chilly for April. The cop at the door told me the parents had arrived home about noon from their winter home in Florida and found their twenty-four-year-old son dead. As the cop is telling me this I'm amazed to see that the house has these flies buzzing in the air. It's those big nasty brutes built like MAC trucks and they are zooming around banging into things.

I think it's not possible; it's too early for flies, it's too cold and they usually don't arrive till a month later. I'm introduced to the middle-aged parents and I tell them I'll look at their son and come and talk with them. The cop leads me down a hallway to a rear bedroom where the doorway is partially open and there is a light on inside. In a room just before this, I stop and stand in awe at one of the most amazing things I have ever seen in the middle of a suburban residence.

The room is stacked on one side with fifty cases of Busch Beer, full, and on the other side are forty-nine cases, empty. I'm still scratching my head as I walk to the last bedroom where those big flies are zooming out. I enter the room and, sitting up in bed across from a TV, is their son, being consumed by maggots mostly visible on face, neck and upper chest. The face, or what is left of it, has a prosthetic eyeball with a lovely blue color staring out at me and I think, my god, now I have finally seen it all. The bed is a hospital bed, very modern, worked electronically, and on the tray table is the fiftieth case of Busch beer, of which thirteen have been consumed within arm's reach of the corpse. I pull back the sheets reluctantly and check to make sure there are no unusual holes or injuries. I don't see any pupa cases and the maggots are getting fat; this indicates the better part of two weeks or more.

I'm amazed to wonder how they even managed to get into the house to do this kind of damage that we usually only see in very warm weather. I tell the cop to call the detectives and the crime scene boys. I go and talk with the parents.

The house still seems cool and the father explains that the chimney is damaged and needs to be repaired. In one of the recent storms about two weeks ago, the wind had blown the aluminum chimney partially off.

They said they had received a call from a neighbor to their house in Florida; they had tried to call their son but got no answer. They arrived home and found him dead. I asked about any medical history that would account for his death.

They told me the following story. Their son, when he was ten years old, was hit by a car while on his bicycle and had multiple fractures and lost his eye. The fractures healed and he got a glass eye but he was never the same child. He got a large award from the insurance company, which was put into an account till he was twenty-one. He never did well in high school and had a lot of trouble and fights over teasing about his fake eye. Girls shunned him. He didn't graduate and spent most of his time in dirtball bars and working low-paying jobs. He had numerous arrests for drunk driving and lost his license and this all got worse when he became twenty-one and had an unlimited income.

Since he was pretty reclusive anyway, they made him a deal. He could drink all he wanted at home and they wouldn't hassle him. It was better than him drinking in those dirtball bars and having to come staggering home. So for the past three years he had spent his days watching TV and drinking beer. The father retired and got a place in Florida for the winter and they had been snow-birding for three years and his son seemed to like that even better. There had been no real problem with this arrangement.

The autopsy showed his death was due to alcoholism and he'd been dead earlier than I thought, probably mid-winter. I learned something about flies: that, attracted by the smell of the corpse, they had found him through the damaged chimney.

Since I am a referential man, I will end with the closing lines of a poem by World War I poet Siegfried Sassoon, the title of which is *Suicide in the Trenches* (for all three of these cases are suicides):

> *'Sneak home and pray you'll never know*
> *The place where youth and laughter go'.*

HERE'S MY HEART

I was awake before the phone rang. It was just a simple pronouncement, not too far away – and in those days, I never needed to write down the address. It was just as well as I wouldn't have gotten back to sleep and it was a lovely night. I look back now and think two things about those days. One, that I never had enough sleep, and second that I loved working at night. I have had some of the sweetest moments of my life in quiet, dark drives back and forth to look at corpses, with my own thoughts and some Steely Dan or Pat Metheny on the tape player after a quick stop for a coffee at 7-11 and a pack of smokes at 3 am.

I was awake because of 'the Dream'. Yes, 'the Dream', and this time it was worse than usual. You would think that a guy who works at the morgue and has seen a couple of thousand people dead in the most horrific ways possible might have a propensity for nightmares. The answer is NO. I have almost never had a corpse dream; in fact I almost never dream any other dream than 'the Dream'. All I get, if it penetrates at all, is fragments of events. If you lived as I did in those days with an average of five hours sleep, you would understand. We hardly ever got to the REM sleep stage, where dreams occur, or stay there very long.

There were only four of us and the county wouldn't pay for any more workers, but the truth is we made a lot of money in overtime, so we bitched but went to the bank after we woke up. I had a pretty heavy load of corpses in my memory banks before I even got to Vietnam. While I was working on the psychiatric wards of National Naval Medical Center, Bethesda, Maryland, I also worked in a civilian hospital in the emergency room and we had one almost every night, from natural or unnatural causes.

With this antecedent, I arrived in Vietnam in August 1968 and was immediately addressing a whole lot of new corpses by the usual ghastly ways of war. The first guy I saw was during a typhoon called Bess and he was outside of the BAS (Battalion Aide Station) lying on the ground along with two others. He had a large jagged hole in his neck, just under the jaw. His eyes were open and he had a look of surprise which I can still see today. The others were less surprised, as most corpses are. Then these images were replaced with shattered legs from mines and all that is remembered is the shrieking. This in turn was replaced by six kids burned by 'Willie Peter' (white phosphorus from our artillery) and my kid had a burning penis which, despite all the treatment, never stopped smouldering, and like a chorus I can hear them all moaning for 'nuc' (water), which is the only word of Vietnamese I remember to this day.

Now 'the Dream', in all fairness, preceded all this, and in those days it was intense because it was fresh and new but as the years proceeded, it seemed as intense because I never had any other dream that I even vaguely remembered.

It's not that it came with any regularity, and to this day I never know what triggers it but it comes two, maybe three times a year; when it comes it leaves me devastated and weeping in its wake.

So you ask what is it that could haunt a man who spends his days and nights with corpses, seeing things that would make, and have made, some men raving maniacs or hopeless drunks? A dream that has appeared unbidden with regularity in someone's life for over thirty years. What could he have seen or done that would bring such a haunting which, given my lifestyle, makes any sense?

Well, the answer is Darlene (Doll), my high school sweetheart. My first love. The dream is always the same. It starts out with us together and I think we're in a park where she went to college after high school. She is on the swings and I am pushing her and she is laughing. This lasts for what seems a short time and then she is gone and the joy is replaced by such a deep feeling of loss and almost physical pain and sadness that it wakes me up. Sometimes after the dream the feeling of wanting to be with her is so bad I get out an old bottle of her perfume I always kept and put some on my pillow. It's called 'Here's My Heart'.

She was the sister of a friend, her older brother who used to work at a boat yard near where I worked. We used to go duck hunting and fishing and drinking. She was my age and we went to the same high school. I was hospitalized with appendicitis and she visited me as a candy stripe nurse (a hospital volunteer). Over the course of my stay, I fell in love with her. She didn't know this and for weeks I was in agony because I was afraid to tell her. One night at a hot dog joint, under the influence or some 'Old Grand-Dad' whiskey, I told her that I loved her. I just said it straight out, and that I understood if she didn't feel the same way. I don't remember now what she said, but, as we left to catch the bus home, she put her arm around me and held me tight as we walked and to this day that one act remains with me, and I long to feel it again.

She was the first woman I ever spent the night with. A chaste night by modern standards but it was the first time as well that I heard birds singing at sunrise as I held her. I never had a sister, just two brothers, and women were a mystery to me.

I almost stabbed some guy at a party we went to, who was paying way too much attention to her and was twice my size, before I was restrained. Thank God.

The few times we had arguments and I thought she was lost to me, I cradled my shotgun, thinking about my loss.

I went into the Navy two weeks after high school graduation and she went to Europe with her parents. I met her after boot camp and she went to a college two hours away from me at Bethesda.

When, I think about it now, I remained a boy and she

wanted a man and it took me a few more years to reach that status. So we broke up in 1966 – March.

So I live with this weird thing in my psyche all these years, thinking I am the only man in the world who gets these strange dreams about lost love. Then, in the space of a few years, I'm astounded to find that I'm not alone.

The movie *Love in the Time of Cholera* left me in a pool of tears, but with a hope that I had barely even thought of or considered.

Is it possible that my Darlene who was nineteen when she met and later married a guy who was twenty-six, would be a widow in the future and I could re-enter her life and we could live the love that should always have been?

I wish her husband a long life but I also wish that I can see her again once before I die. When I saw that movie, I thought some guy had just written a fantasy – and then I saw *The Reader* and I have never been the same since.

Whatever *Love in the Time of Cholera* was about, my feelings were more like the main character, played by my favourite actor Ralph Fiennes. Maybe men should never think of themselves as this vulnerable but I always have. This movie has the intensity and drama of every dream I have ever had about my beloved Doll. The fact that he would wreck his whole emotional life for this love doesn't matter. I did the same thing myself. The memory of that arm around me on a night long ago haunts me still.

When it comes to Darlene I'm still a boy. If I were a man I should have recognized and understood what is evident now. I never have any bad dreams. I spent most of this story complaining about that, when I should have been thanking the stars and the gods or just plain good fortune or luck, considering what I've seen and done. The collective misery and horror of seeing 30,000 dead people has never intruded into my psyche other than the pain I still feel forty years later from the loss of my own happiness. The appalling realization of this level of egotism/narcissism you might think borders on the psychopathic – and, having been in psychiatry, I'm inclined to agree with you.

I like to think that, considering the price I should/could pay for having to deal with this level of inhumanity and sadness which in part is a consequence of that loss, that 'the Dream' has protected me all these years and still does. Call it a life jacket that I have clung to in a sea of misery, or a bullet-proof vest for a heart too vulnerable.

It also, considering how numbing the trauma of seeing all this death can be, has left me with the one emotion I need for repair. LOVE.

There is a wonderful song by Little Anthony and the Imperials called *The Wonder of it All*. I like this part best. Little Anthony got what I felt about her perfectly. So, with slight modification:

Love at last had found me
And put her arm around me.
I can't explain what I feel,
But I feel like a king,
Now, that I had your love.
I'm not alone, now that we're one.'

Thanks, Doll, for my 'Sweet Dream'
Love always,
JACK

THE EMPATH

As if it wasn't already a bad week for lots of reasons (reasons anyone reading the preceding stories might have a pretty good clue about), I had another one of 'THEM'. I hate 'THEM' almost more than corpses covered in maggots. 'What is THEM?' you ask.

Well in the original *Star Trek* series there was an episode about the 'empath'. Kirk and Spock are captured by aliens (what else?) and wind up in some kind of zoo where these big-headed guys called the Viands (which is Anglo-French for food) are trying to see how humans and other species will react to various things, but mostly torture.

In this zoo is a lovely woman called an 'empath', whose species has the unique trait of absorbing pain. It's never made clear if there are men empaths or children empaths or if they absorb pain of any species or just humans in particular. What's also not explained is how empaths feel between absorptions. If you're dead can you absorb vibes of pain? Hey, they're aliens, everyone knows they can do anything. Kirk gets tortured again and the empath heals him almost to the point of her death.

When I first saw this, I thought here it is, this is me. This is what I do for a living, have always done for a living. I go and absorb pain. So now I'll tell you about 'THEM'.

At least once or twice a year I go to a lovely home in a quiet neighborhood to find the owner dead. Not only is the owner dead (they are always men) but one of the first things you see is a sign on a wall or on a table that says 'in case of emergency'. There you find, neatly laid out, the names and addresses of family, friends or executors, as well as physicians and the name of a local funeral home. Legal documents and just about everything anyone dealing with the dead will need in order to get the family notified and the body to a funeral home or crematorium.

The houses are typically the oldest on the block and, although usually well-maintained, need work. Some of them are in declining neighborhoods, places that were once more affluent. Inside there is old furniture, usually on the dark wood side, and sagging couches. The main feature is an overwhelming desiccated fetid smell of dust and dryness.

Most times they are dead in bed or in a chair, usually fully-dressed and always clean-shaved. The alarm clocks always say 5 am. They are on the floor, occasionally decomposed but dry, almost mummified.

This fellow today is unusual as he's up on the head of the bed, leaning against a window covered in plastic, probably trying to get a breath while gasping perhaps. The house was locked (the cops broke in); his wallet is in his pants and no unusual injuries. He's eighty-seven years old. He has a black-and-white TV, a Dumont, and on his bookshelves are *Reader's Digest* condensed books from the '50s. I read many of these as a kid. My favorite was *Century of the Surgeon*.

There are family photographs going back generations and it looks like he has a lot of grandchildren. There is also, on a wall in the den, a certificate for a silver star won in World War I. He killed a German machine gun crew in a place called Fismes in France in October 1918. Old suits in the closet, bathroom fixtures ancient but still solid.

It's hard to tell how long he's been waiting. I hear the Beatles singing *Eleanor Rigby* in the background as I go from room to room: 'All the lonely people, where do they all belong?' The wife has been gone a good long while, I guess, from the look of the place. Neighbors see him now and then. He stopped driving a few years ago after a minor accident and stopped going to church as well. All of 'THEM' are always skinny and usually have a few bottles of stuff no one drinks any more but were staples when I was a kid. Rock & Rye, Fleishman's whiskey, Black and White scotch, Tangery gin.

It's just so fucking sad and, being an 'empath', I absorb it all. Alone in an empty house, 'killing time, till time kills you', like a big sand-dial filling the room inexorably with all the seconds, minutes, hours, days, weeks, months, years, decades, until the weight of all this time crushes the life out of you. When I was a kid, one of the greatest movies I ever saw was called the *Incredible Shrinking Man* – who, after exposure to atomic fallout, starts to shrink and ultimately shrinks into atoms. See, as an 'empath', I know this is going to be my fate.

I get beeped while absorbing pain. I call the office. It's a kid with cancer who died at home. I wonder if it's possible that, like the 'empath', I'm living on an alien planet and I'm employed by the Viands? They pay pretty good but there is too much pain on this planet with humans. The idea of a planet of empaths somewhere who don't actually inflict pain on each other, knowing how much it hurts, and that someday I might go there is a far better idea than anything going on in the land of the free and home of the brave.

CURIOSITY

Curiosity, you would think, would be one of the most essential ingredients in anyone who claims or wants to be in this business. Yet curiosity is not an essential ingredient as it turns out.

So what is curiosity? Why do some of us have it and others less and where does it come from? As it turns out it's a rather curious trait.

In fact there is almost no evidence of anyone every trying to figure it out. Don't believe me, 'Google' it and see what you can find? The one theory that I found years ago without the internet comes from a woman psychiatrist. One of the great women psychiatrists who came after Anna Freud, like Melanie Klein who concerned themselves with women's and children's psychiatric issues in the *Dawn of Modern Psychiatry*. As far as I know no other psychiatrist has commented on the origins of curiosity.

The theory goes something like this. The newborn infant whose whole early life revolves around issues of eating and comfort will, after a while, come to the sense that it knows its environment. When it is not being handled or asleep or being fed, it lays there absorbing sensations. Sounds and things that pass within its vision. It knows when it's being handled but it develops its own ideas about what's going on when it's not being stimulated by caregivers or family members. It sees, but mostly it listens.

Psychiatry in its infancy placed a heavy sense on early psychological exposure to sexuality of adults. Freud later had to suppress this idea because it was turning people off who thought his work valuable in other areas. His theory that children were traumatized by the primal scene of 'parents having sex' when families lived all together in single rooms under trying conditions, gave way to a more modern idea where the infant in the same room would hear parents engaged in passion and mistake it for violence like seeing the event as well.

As the 20th century progressed and children were banished to the nursery or their own rooms, this led the infant left alone to wonder where the caregiver was who cared for it. All of these issues according to this lady psychiatrist gives rise to the infant who feels need, and wants to know why it's not being attended to and being left alone. That's it right or wrong.

I've thought about this and added my own thoughts about the whole business. If you have good parents and they meet your every need with regularity then the infant has no need to wonder. I think the infant who has less assured parenting is left to come to another sense and its sense, maybe even anxiety, is stimulated to try to understand. In Freud's day, in pre birth control days, families were large and mothers had little time for the kind of childcare we have today with smaller families.

Sorry to have taken you down this road but as it turns out the lady psychiatrist who has been the only one to comment on curiosity, lived in the town where I presently reside. Curious is it not?

In fact a place named after her is not far from where I and my new wife live in an apartment over a photography shop where there are still gas jet lamps that work on the main street. Even more to her credit, they offer low cost psychiatric care which is a rarity in the county, country.

As it turns out our apartment is part of a series of apartments over store fronts and the rear windows open onto a courtyard which the shop owners can use, but we can hear everything.

It's pretty quiet back there with one exception. This particular place is occupied by a bantam-sized man with a shock of white hair who is not surprisingly known as 'Whitey', whose main occupation seems to be drinking and wife slugging. We would hear this periodically from our windows especially in summer. Occasionally cops would arrive as well. 'Whitey' had a son who was the spitting image of him and also had white hair as a boy. Those apartments were ovens in summer and you'd see 'Whitey' and son outside on the steps. Sullen.

Well, that clinic I told you about which was near my house was in a lovely mock Tudor wooden building which was part of an office complex of four structures. One was used by my attorney. One night the clinic that was named after the lady psychiatrist burnt to the ground and the fire department worked hard to save the others.

It turns out the fire was started by 'Whitey's' son who was under treatment at the clinic named after the famous psychiatrist. I don't have to be curious to figure out why he would do that. Whatever they were saying to him, they weren't stopping 'Whitey' Sr from drinking and slugging his wife and 'Whitey' Jr was maybe ten years old.

At the time I thought, having spent many years in psychiatry, that the kid had got it right. No one was helping him stop his crazy father, not police, or shrinks. After the fire they surely paid attention. Hope 'Whitey' Jr had a better life but the odds are against it, but I would be curious to know.

BODY BAGS

It's another day, it's early morning and I am with my lovely twin baby girls who are two years old. They are having their usual morning romp on these little plastic vehicles that look like shoes and they zoom around the house. I chase them, making ominous noises, feign inability to catch them, while they shriek and laugh. All this is precious to a man who has spent his night on various mayhems, horrors and disasters to earn his daily bread in forensic medicine.

Maybe, if I had never been in psychiatry, Vietnam, or surgery, I might be having difficulty in being able to do this without either intruding into the reality of the other. They say that sociopaths have the curious ability to kill and feel no emotion, but I just can't ever feel anything but 'Emotion' and, unlike the rest of the medical profession of which I so much want to be a part of, I have never been able or have developed that ability to witness horrific things without it intruding on my equanimity at least half the time. It's beginning to bother me less and less that I have these two images in my mind.

Robert J. Lifton MD, a psychiatrist who wrote a book called *Home from the War*, about the Vietnam war, says doctors developed an ability he calls 'Doubling' to deal with stressful issues and not have it intrude into their private lives. Physicians should feel the pain of every decision they make for good or bad if they claim to have any legitimate right to care for humanity.

We used to have a saying in Vietnam: 'Don't mean nothing'. This was to explain missing platoon members whose disappearance we had either witnessed or not. Yet, I now noticed that I had developed the curious habit of seeing things but not letting them intrude on my psyche too much, no matter how bad it had been. It's not that I couldn't tell you in minute detail how events had occurred, it's just that they had no emotional register after a day or two. 'Don't mean nothing' is really the perfect Vietnam metaphor as psychiatrically it is a 'dissociative statement' and the first step to sociopathy as well as 'Doubling'. We all acquired it as a common denominator for survival in the Marine Corps in Vietnam back in 1968. I wasn't aware how easily I had slipped back into the mindset until I was back from Vietnam and witnessed some of the same things in civilian life.

Once, coming back from vacation in Maine to see my old Navy buddy, Shep Chase, I came across a head-on collision on route 495 in Massachusetts. Fresh bodies thrown out, some hanging dead from windows and in a flash I was out and running across the median. But there was only one survivor, a young girl with two broken arms who was seated next to her dead mother, whose whole body was in the space where your feet go to touch the pedals. This young girl had her hands hanging down at 45 degree angles from mid forearm fractures. An ambulance showed up and out came a nurse completely dressed in white; cap and shoes included. She didn't want to walk into the pool of motor oil I was standing in so I asked her for splints and did the job for her. I then carried the girl to the edge of the oil and onto a stretcher, telling her all the time her mother was OK and would follow shortly. The look on my wife's face after I came back, hands and clothing covered in blood, said it all.

Another time, driving to work for an 8 am OR case where I was assisting, I came across another accident. A man whose car had a flat tire on the highway had gotten out and walked to the rear of his car to get the spare tire when a group of High School students, who had been out all night after their senior prom, rammed into the back of his car. There he was sitting on the hood of the other car, both legs almost off, blood pouring out, white in shock and people standing around. I jumped up on cars giving orders and made two tourniquets from belts – mine and another man's – and got some guys to pull the cars back. We moved him to a small hillside nearby, his head down for shock purposes. I was wrapping his legs when one of the fractured bones lacerated my hand, but I got them wrapped and finally rescue arrived. However, instead of hauling ass to a nearby hospital, they spent twenty minutes trying to start an IV (wouldn't let me) before they gave up and rolled. I had time to get the ER doc at the hospital where I worked to stitch my hand before I got to the OR to scrub. I did the case with an extra glove on my injured hand. No one really believed my story till next day when there was a report in the newspapers.

So, after a couple of years at the morgue, it was seamless. I was perfectly at ease at 8 am with my kids after pulling corpses into bags at 4 am. The incongruity of it all never seemed to matter as long as the two worlds were separate. In fact, one gave more poignancy to the other. After a while I stopped thinking about it and just accepted the 'Doubling' world, so maybe Dr Lifton is right but I knew deep down inside that soon or later hanging around all this death would get to me.

You pay the price for this. You see things you wish you never had. It would be better to have your eyes plucked out like in some ancient Greek myth. You find out things, just knowing it will cause your psyche to repress it so deeply in your unconscious mind that a thousand years of psychotherapy will never bring it to consciousness.

It was very simple work really, just like Vietnam (better than Vietnam, no danger and pay so much better) as I'd be out all night attending suicides, cancer patients, heart attacks and car wrecks where there would be red flares smoking, flashing lights, grim-faced men in uniform, camera strobe lights, guns, blood, twisted metal, burning oil and, of course, mangled corpses; all leading to body bags.

Sometimes after a bad night I would go to a topless bar near the office and see the lovely ladies dancing nude after all this death, just to get an injection of humanity. I used to think of myself as the 'Grim Reaper' because they are not dead until I say they are (that's why the cops need me) or Charon who would cart them off to the Hades (morgue). There we then cut them open (modern autopsy) and cut parts of them into little pieces to see in microcosm what we saw in macrocosm. It's like having the job which is now very popular called the 'Cleaner', following a serial killer, always having to clean up after him and amazed at the choices he was making.

The thing that saved me, I like to think, was the hours I spent every day with my babies. It's nuts you say, but believe me that child care made almost all the bad stuff go away and maybe Robert J. Lifton MD, who has never espoused any alternative for what he calls 'Doubling', might be glad knowing that the nurturing joy that few men ever get to understand and leave mostly to their wives, saved my life and for that I will always be grateful to my lovely daughters.

BRAIN DEAD

I f my life was a movie, and there are days when I think it should be and days where I'm convinced it really is, this would be the part where the main character (me) has one of those flashbacks that adds life, tragedy or poignancy to the character's travails. I don't know at what point in his telling me (the intern from the hospital) that the patient had met all the 'Brain Death' criteria and been pronounced dead that the flashback occurred.

Maybe it was the matter of fact tone in his voice as he reeled off the criteria, which he probably just learned from attending this particular patient's death. Maybe he thought as those hospital docs usually do, that he was the big professor telling a lowly investigator at the Medical Examiner's office the things the smart guys know. Maybe he needed to reel it off to convince himself what he just witnessed and participated in was legal, fair and moral to the Medical Examiner as some kind of absolution.

It would be a nice voiceover for the beginning of the flashback, like the beginning of a Raymond Chandler short story. As the scene dissolves maybe a date would flash up like the actual date 1977 on the screen. The dissolve in this case would show a young man with a full head of dark brown hair dressed in green OR scrubs being spoken to by a similarly dressed older surgeon. He says to the young man, 'I know it's been a long day in the OR for you but there is a surgeon coming from the Organ Donor Program at the County Medical Center and he needs some help taking the kidneys for donation from a brain injured patient in ICU whose just been pronounced brain dead.'

The young man (me), who is the surgeon's assistant, looks aghast and says, 'That he has no experience removing kidneys since we are general and vascular surgeons.'

The older man says with a smile that he can do it and that he should just do what the other surgeon tells him and off he goes. The young man calls his wife to say he will be late again and hears again the anger and disappointment in her voice.

He drifts into the nearby ICU and looks at the patient who he has known about since his admission. It was a small ICU then, seven beds, and the others were filled with his patients. It's hard to see the patient's face as he has an endo-tracheal tube in place connected to a respirator and a Levin tube in his nose and the tape used to hold these in place covers most of the face. He's a tall man with a well built, muscular body, lithe almost and dirty blond hair, lots of it. The story the ICU nurses had told him was that he had been celebrating his daughter's birthday, he had been drinking heavily and that he had blown out an aneurysm in his brain ten days before. No

CAT scans in those days. Angiogram confirmed the diagnosis and that, plus the new criteria for brain death, would make this young man one of the first to be pronounced 'Brain Dead' and have his kidneys removed for donation. The criteria included back then negative EEGs (electro-encephalo-graphs), absent corneal reflexes and other cerebellar reflexes and apnea off the respirator. His heart was still beating, his blood pressure was being artificially elevated and his kidneys were making urine.

The nurses seemed uneasy about all this as we all did back then. We knew that a step had been taken into some new place in the advance of medicine and that this wasn't a good thing to be part of. Mother Nature doing her job was one thing, but turning off life-saving devices wasn't one of them. We spent a lot of time putting those devices in.

It's not that I hadn't seen things with terminally ill cancer patients getting morphine every four hours whether they needed it or not, till they died. Once on grand rounds on a pediatric ward a big discussion was taking place about an infant born with Down's Syndrome and an intestinal ailment (duodenal atresia) that needed surgery but the family didn't want to give consent. The discussion finally led to the hospital deciding that its job was to save people not to help them die and the infant was sent home to die, with his unconsenting parents watching.

In those days there wasn't as much monetary pressure as there is today... Medicare and Medicaid provided lots of long-term bill paying. The kidney transplant business was now becoming more common with the discovery of new drugs to stop the rejection problem, but this was still a very rare business.

When I think of it now, that older surgeon, my boss, was also Chief of Surgery at the hospital where we worked. He could have asked any of the urology staff or about two dozen other surgeons on staff to help remove those kidneys. He could have asked one of the five other surgeons in our own surgical group or done it himself, but he didn't. He asked his surgical assistant because I realize now no one wanted to have any part in this 'Brain Death' business. So they gave it to me who was too dumb to understand perhaps how they felt or indeed refuse because I looked at my boss and others as GODS and would do anything they asked to be part of what they did, which was saving lives and fighting disease.

I hung around the OR lounge smoking and reading a medical journal till the surgeon arrived. He was a young guy, a few years older than me. I got him set up and they wheeled the patient in. It was quiet in the OR as it was now after regular hours. The gas man didn't know if he was to use any pain drugs other than the muscle relaxants.

The surgery was more like an autopsy and kidneys are harder to remove from a supine position. We cut his abdomen into four quarters vertically and horizontally. The kidneys turned out to be the easier part of the procedure. Taking out the ureters was much harder. After a while it got to be pretty bloody as we weren't tying off the small bleeders as normal because the kidneys had to be taken out quickly and flushed in iced saline and packed in ice before being rushed off for transplant at other hospitals. Suffice to say we tied off major blood vessels but it was pretty much a lake of blood when we finished. We closed the abdomen very simply and the gas man turned off the respirator with reluctance. We all walked away while the heart was still beating; you could see it on the monitor and feel a weak pulse. I had a sick feeling inside along with the pride that the young doctor had thanked me for helping him. He said I had good hands which is probably the best compliment you can give to any surgeon.

I wandered back to ICU to get some coffee and have a smoke in the nurses' lounge area. The dead man's chart was brought back from the OR. I looked at the man's name again and saw that he lived in the town where I went to high school and that we were the same age. I thought, that's funny and then the name exploded in my head – 'I KNEW THIS GUY'. It was twelve years after graduation but I knew who he was and he knew me. We traveled in the same semi-hoodlum working class, non-academic or college bound groups. He was a handsome boy, well loved by the girls and a bit of a wild man. When I got home I looked in my high school year book. I saw his picture but he hadn't signed it. We weren't that close thank GOD.

Dissolve back to modern time. I tell the intern thanks, I'll take care of it from here and send the body to the morgue for us to pick and and write my report.

If I was Raymond Chandler's Marlowe, this is where I'd reach in my desk for the bottle of RYE and pour a healthy dose, light up a smoke and lean back in my chair and watch the flies buzzing about the office.

Since I'm me, I think of the lines:

That this is what we fear
No sight, no sound, no touch
Taste or smell
Nothing to think with
Nothing to look or link with
The anaesthetic from which none come round

Aubade by Phillip Larkin

COURAGE

I arrive in the late afternoon sun which shows off the brickwork of yellow stone at its best. The façade has held up well for almost a hundred-plus years. The original stone runners of the three entrance steps have been replaced, but the old bed and side walls, as well as the two lampposts, are still intact as a photo of Dr Rivers standing in front of the place shows very clearly. There are benches to sit on but the once spectacular views have been lost to trees now and there is not much to contemplate as I sit. There are eighteen disabled parking places at the entrance drive, but it is not an entrance any more but the rear of a huge alien spaceship building that has been grafted onto the back of this 'Old Hydro'/Dottyville of renown.

I wonder, could you get a disabled sticker for shellshock? Neurasthenia surely? I imagine Sassoon's and Owen's cars parked outside. It's not as far fetched as these parking places (at least in the USA), always blue in color as it is the sign you have in your car. Blue armbands had to be worn while off site by officer patients.

I have a fondness for places like this, old buildings that once housed the metally ill. In 1966, I became a Neuro-psychiatric technician at the National Naval Medical Center, Bethesda,

Maryland. Code number 8485 as all Navy job skills are so designated with code numbers. The most dreaded was the 8404 which was the one you got before you went to Vietnam. I got mine two years later.

Freshly minted after four months' training in all aspects of modern psychiatric care, which also included a two week stint at St Elisabeth's hospital in DC where Ezra Pound had been a patient for over ten years much like Sassoon for his political utterances as opposed to his psychiatric state.

There was no poetry and no poets on my short visit. To those who have read *One Flew Over thè Cuckoo's Nest*, the book describes what it looked like to a T.

Bethesda Neuro-psychiatric wards comprised one whole six-story building (called building 7 for some reason) grafted on much like modern Craiglockhardt to an earlier structure of the 1930's hospital. It had no bars on the windows but heavy screens covered most windows.

All the wards were exactly same in basic design' forty-five bed capacity in each. 7B was the Neurology ward. 7C was the enlisted men's open ward where patients could come and go and get liberty and leave as they recovered and awaited new orders. 7D was the enlisted men's closed ward (we never said locked but it was) this was where you were admitted initially and treated till you went down to 7C. 7E was the female ward. Half of the ward was closed (locked) and was made up mostly of active duty women and wives and daughters of active duty enlisted men and officers. 7F was the officer ward the same as 7E, half (closed) and a mix of active and retired officers.

We had some great psychiatrists who were much admired. Colorful men who had learned their skills in World War II and Korea. The daytime business of psychiatric care revolves around meals, medications, medical tests, occupational therapy, group therapy and individual psychiatric therapy much as Owen and Sassoon would have had with Rivers and Brock. After dinner in the evening there would be TV, radio and cards; endless games of cards. Lights out at 9.30 following sleep meds being handed out.

Unlike Craiglockhardt we had no shellshock cases other than one marine who had broken down under heavy shelling near the DMZ (mostly because the enemy had no artillery other than near DMZ) and had rapidly recovered, even before arriving at our hospital.

Our daily work was dealing with the pernicious effects of the conscription and recruiters and recruits anxious to stay out of the Army. So we were confronted mostly with men unfit for military service for various psychiatric reasons who broke down in the first year of service mostly.

The officer wards were populated mostly by elderly officers with dementia and the usual problems of Navy officers at sea (alcohol and depression) for hundreds of years as opposed to war in Vietnam and even these were few as they were career men and tough. It was always disconcerting to me anyway to have to give orders to officers saying, 'Admiral it's time for occupational therapy' and march him off.

It's hard to say now but the women's ward was mostly filled with serving women who had problems in a man's Navy. The duties on this ward were shared by Navy Corps Waves and corpsmen. The biggest taboo and problem was these young women were very attractive and seductive. Sooner or later a neuro-psychiatric technician would have sex relations with the psychiatric female patient and almost invariably she would tell her doctor.

I spent most of my time on enlisted wards and was later Senior Corpsman of Neurology ward. You want war trauma big time. Be a twenty-year-old third class hospital corpsman in charge of a ward at The National Naval Medical Center, Bethesda, Maryland, outside of Washington DC in wartime, and see the Captain of the Psychiatric service and the Chief Nurse, who was a full three-stripe Naval Commander, getting off the elevator outside your ward ready for the monthly white glove inspection, then you will know FEAR.

I never saw nor did any of those smart Psychiatrists see anything that later became PTSD. I think now that all the suffering of veterans post-war in two world wars and Korea, was considered normal as long as you functioned mostly and got on with life. The majority of Vietnam veterans returned home and got on with their lives like our fathers and grandfathers, happy to be alive despite 'ugly thoughts' as Siegfried called them.

I've come to this place to see a play called *Not About Heroes* and the title makes me ill until I see that it's a phrase used by Owen in his famous preface and, like poppy, overused to this day.

Sassoon says in the introduction to the first publication of Owen's poems the following: 'All that was strongest in Wildred Owen survives in his poems: any superficial impressions of his personality, any records of his conversations, behavior or appearance would be irrelevant and unseemly. The curiosity which demands such morsels would be incapable of appreciating the richness of his work.' I wonder if the author or actors have read Sassoon's words and see this as a warning; it clearly seems to not stage Owen's life anyway.

The play is staged in the Sassoon room of the Rivers Suite at Craiglockhardt. It's a big room at ground level and both rooms (the other Owen's) were probably the communal dining rooms which, just like a Bethesda, the patients ate with the staff.

I'm not, and should never be thought of as, a theatre critic. The two young actors are very good and the chap who plays Owen looks remarkably like him. The script is made from published remarks and letters of both of these men. I know what they have said, but in this setting and seeing it actually being reproduced, well, let's just say my mind wanders. I think how as I hear their words and know their predicament that I've been down this road myself.

In November 1968 (fifty years later a week after the day Owen was killed) I had been wounded by our own ammunition and spent ten days in hospital then back I went, anxious to get back to my platoon responsibilites. No one wants a sick or wounded corpsman especially himself. No fine words or anything even close to these fine poets contemplating their returns. Vietnam was where the term 'Wasted' became how we described our deaths. There was no poetry although I could have read and felt at home with Owen's and Sassoon's works, but wars are fought by ignorant youth and no one was more ignorant at the age of twenty-one, my fourth year in the Navy. The title of one of the first and few books about Vietnam was *If I Die in a Combat Zone: Box Me Up and Ship Me Home* by Tim O'Brien. Hardly as edifying a title as *Anthem for Doomed Youth* or *Dulce et Decorum Est*, although what's described in both poems was true in my time as well.

Being in a combat zone is like being on death row, you're not sure if you're going to get a reprieve and every day you have to keep that idea out of your mind. I learned from *If I Die in a Combat Zone* the following, and I think what I'm seeing and hearing in this play and their words is the same.

Plato said courage is one of four parts of virtue. It is there with temperance, justice and wisdom, and all parts are necessary to make a sublime human being. He also says men without courage are men without justice, temperance or wisdom, just as without wisdom, men are not truly courageous. Men must know what they do is courageous, they must know it is right and that kind of knowledge is wisdom and nothing else which is why I know few brave men. Either they are stupid and do not know what is right, or they know what is right and can't bring themselves to do it knowing the likely consequences, or they know what is right and do not feel and understand the fear that must be overcome. It takes a special man. They have all the parts. Sassoon and Owen have temperance and wisdom from previous battles, they know it's right to return and they know the fear which they have to overcome and sadly the consequences. Two sublime men.

Wilfred probably wrote his famous preface about heroes in ignorance of what Siegfried wrote on 24 August 1917 as he had only met him on the 22nd. Siegfried probably didn't show Wilfred but on that day he received the news of the death of Stephen Gordon Harboard, a fox hunting friend of his youth, near Ypres. He wrote one of his bitterest war poems *The Wooden Cross*, which is a poetic epitaph for that friend. Not knowing of the preface Owen would write it became Owen's epitaph as well.

The world's too full of heroes, mostly dead
Mocked by rich wreaths and words nobly said
And it's no gain to you nor mend our loss
To know that you've earned a glorious wooden cross

Siegfried also wrote a review of this play and it's from *Siegfried's Journey*:

Once in his lifetime, perhaps, a man may be the instrument through which something constructive emerges, whether it be genius giving birth to an original idea or the anonymous mortal who makes the most of an opportunity that will never recur. It is for the anonymous ones that I have my special feeling. I like to think of them remembering the one time when they were involved in something unusual or important - when, probably without knowing it at the time, they, as it were, wrote their single masterpiece, never to perform anything comparable again. Then they were fully alive, living above themselves, and discovering powers they hadn't been aware of. For a moment they stood in the transfiguring light of dramatic experience...

Strange, I think, to be in an earlier version of a place where I spent my youth like theirs in wartime and stranger still that they both never saw the poetry of pity and compassion that led me to care for the sick and the injured in war. I had never thought then and for many years after to write a poem about all this suffering that I had witnessed, yet they so readily were able to do so.

POEMS

THE JOB

Eyeball flat and stuck on a wood deck
Almost missed in all the seagull dreck.
Dead owner, a young man twenty feet away
Empty shotgun points the way.

Half a glass of Chivas and Schweppes to steel
The trembling hands soon not to feel.
Furrowed skull blown open to sight
Fifteen day maggots frolic in delight.

Afternoon sun reaches this place
Lightens obscenely the decomposed face.
Others look away, but I'm paid to see
I'm the modern day, Charon, that's me.

Eyeball in hand, I pause to go
I think I should have some feeling, but no
Emotion needs to be spread
It's just two guys who are dead.

MORGUE WAGON

Driving with Jimmy in a corpse filled truck
Five am, smoking Lucky Strikes, don't give a fuck.
A suicide, a wreck, a double murder, a crazy
It's been a long summer night and I'm a little hazy.

Bugs smash the windshield and splatter
The windshield never washed but no matter.
Wonderful dawn starting to show
Golden rays coming into view, three hours to go.

Bring out your dead, I yell on Main street
Driving to a diner to get something to eat.
Blood on my hands and on my clothes
The smell of death is in my nose.

It gets so that sometimes I'm afraid
That no emotion is shown or displayed.
Jimmy never has any fear, he says
He has lived many more of these days.

So, I hope that he's right and fear will go
I'll have to continue doing this to know.
Bugs smash the windshield and splatter.
Windshield never washed. Does it matter?

11 PM

I see the body from the door
Old man lying on the basement floor.
Red halo surrounds your broken visage
like a Russian icon image.

Blood streaked across the floor
As you tried to drag yourself to the door.
Fractured leg and bleeding head
It took awhile to be dead.

13 steps to solid concrete
Worn place on the step for aged feet.
Bannister wrongly placed for it
Arthritic hand too weak to fit.

Basement shelves filled with toys
For children who are no longer girls or boys.
The kids pleaded with you not to live alone
But you didn't want to leave your home.

So now your fate is the concrete floor
Only a couple of feet from the door.
No one came to help you out
Did you die with a whimper or a shout?

PRONOUNCEMENT

Now! I've pronounced you dead.
It's all done but not said.
Old man, white-haired, peaceful still.
Sun shining in clear and
Clean at the sill.

I have met and unmet you.
Seeing but not seen by you.
Touching but not touched by you.
Remembering I hope nothing of you.

You and hundreds of others have
Made me so unable to think of a
Future beyond today.
Pronouncing you dead makes me
Think of when it will be my time to go.

Old man, you made it easy for me.
I was afraid and now I see.
There is nothing to fear, just
Courage to be. Pronouncing
People dead till it's me.